Non-Representational Geographies of Therapeutic Art Making

Candice P. Boyd

Non-Representational Geographies of Therapeutic Art Making

Thinking Through Practice

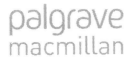

Candice P. Boyd
School of Geography
University of Melbourne
Melbourne, Australia

ISBN 978-3-319-46285-1   ISBN 978-3-319-46286-8 (eBook)
DOI 10.1007/978-3-319-46286-8

Library of Congress Control Number: 2016954082

© The Editor(s) (if applicable) and The Author(s) 2017
This book was advertised with a copyright holder in the name of the publisher in error,
whereas the author holds the copyright.
This work is subject to copyright. All rights are solely and exclusively licensed by the Publisher,
whether the whole or part of the material is concerned, specifically the rights of translation,
reprinting, reuse of illustrations, recitation, broadcasting, reproduction on microfilms or in
any other physical way, and transmission or information storage and retrieval, electronic
adaptation, computer software, or by similar or dissimilar methodology now known or here-
after developed.
The use of general descriptive names, registered names, trademarks, service marks, etc. in this
publication does not imply, even in the absence of a specific statement, that such names are
exempt from the relevant protective laws and regulations and therefore free for general use.
The publisher, the authors and the editors are safe to assume that the advice and information
in this book are believed to be true and accurate at the date of publication. Neither the
publisher nor the authors or the editors give a warranty, express or implied, with respect to
the material contained herein or for any errors or omissions that may have been made.

Cover illustration: Pattern adapted from an Indian cotton print produced in the 19th century

Printed on acid-free paper

This Palgrave Macmillan imprint is published by Springer Nature
The registered company is Springer International Publishing AG
The registered company address is: Gewerbestrasse 11, 6330 Cham, Switzerland

Dedicated to David Bissell—for understanding so completely

PREFACE

This book is based on a five-year engagement with the concepts and ideas of non-representational theory – a pursuit made possible by a supportive partner with a full-time job, my own relatively secure part-time employment as an academic (for most of its duration), an only child who gives and takes in equal measure, and my Australian citizenship.

I came to cultural geography via a pathway of academic research and teaching in clinical psychology, which is not the usual route for a cultural geographer. Unlike many personal journeys, I can trace the starting point back to a specific event. At a point in my career where I was heavily engaged in a programme of research on rural adolescent mental health, John McDonald, a sociologist in the department where I worked, placed a journal article in my mailbox. The article, co-authored by social and cultural geographers Hester Parr and Chris Philo, tackled the topic of rural mental health and the social geographies of caring. In my 10 years as a psychology academic, I had never heard of social and cultural geography. I remember reading the paper and being positively gripped by the explanatory power of the ideas.

Compelled by the corpus of Hester's work, as outlined in her book *Mental Health and Social Space*, I undertook a second PhD in human geography and the creative arts from 2010 to 2015. Based on my research background and expertise, I had always envisaged that the research project would be qualitative. I was a 'seasoned practitioner'. I had 'skills' in listening to people. I had spent years developing expertise in qualitative research methods that flew in the face of psychology's entrenched positivist paradigm, and these skills were hard-won. In the first year of the PhD, however, I read the early work of another cultural geographer, J-D Dewsbury, and was forced to think again.

viii PREFACE

What do we learn by witnessing the world as it unfolds? How might we extend what counts as knowledge by developing an attunement to the world's 'happenings'? How are environments produced, sensed, and performed? What is the status of the human subject in relation to a world that simply 'takes place'? As these questions began to permeate my thinking, I imagined a project that involved working alongside people, observing their practice rather than talking to them about it – engaging with them in *acts of doing* rather than just asking and listening. In a radical change of research direction, I proposed a performative research project to my PhD supervisor, Rachel Hughes, who, in her effortlessly enabling style, embraced the challenge wholeheartedly. I cannot thank her enough for her open-hearted willingness to engage in a process of mutual discovery and invention that, at its completion, rendered me an artist-geographer.

By way of artistic learning, I am most grateful to Magali Gentric and Jason Waterhouse, co-owners and directors of Stockroom in Kyneton, Victoria (Australia). It was through them, and their avid commitment to contemporary art practice, that I was exposed to countless examples of excellent art. Over four years of arduous work, they organised exhibitions that did our rural community great credit. By bringing the city 'up north' and believing that there would be people 'up here' willing and able to receive it, they provided inspiration to many local artists, creators, and collectors. Via the Stockroom and Platform Art Spaces, I also met Kent Wilson and Lucy James – two extraordinary artists whose written, curatorial, sculptural, and visual art practices will always set the bar for me.

As for geographers (in all their guises), 'generosity of spirit' would be a good phrase to describe the vast majority of them. Apart from Rachel and Hester, I am most indebted to Thomas Jellis, Joe Gerlach, and Derek P. McCormack for their advice on my early research direction. David Bissell, Maria Hynes, and Scott Sharpe organised IAG mini-conferences that somehow incisively corresponded to each year of my candidature. Michelle Duffy, Bradley L. Garrett, Martin Zebracki, Harriet Hawkins, Adeline Tay, Irfan Yusuf, Carlo Morris, Tina Richardson, Anja Kanngieser, David Bissell, Theresa Harada, Dean Merlino, Claudia Demichelis, Andrew Gorman-Murray, Sarah Bennett, Pompeo Martelli, Paul Harrison, Alex Cullen, Michael Gallagher, Ruth Raynor, and James Ash have, along with so many others, become colleagues and fine friends. Michelle Duffy, in particular, had enough faith to collaborate with me on several research projects and presentations throughout my candidature. Thanks also to Andrew Lapworth and Tom Roberts for their collegiality at the 2012 AAG Meeting in New York.

I would also like to acknowledge Chris Philo, Hayden Lorimer, Eric Laurier, and Derek P. McCormack for making time for me to interview them during a three-week visit to the UK in 2011. Despite their busy working schedules, each of them gave an hour of their time to openly share their thoughts on non-representational theory as I audio-recorded them. Further to this, I had the privilege during my first London RGS-IBG conference in 2012 to attend a session on geography and post-phenomenology convened by James Ash and Paul Simpson. I have since witnessed, with pleasure, the development of their stimulating paper from manuscript to publication. From there, I screened my short film *Sound as Ekphrasis* at the Nordic Geographers' Meeting in Reykjavík in 2013 which was incidentally attended by Matthew Shepherd, a PhD student from the University of Oxford. Matthew later travelled to Melbourne to co-convene a seminar on practice-based methods in geography and provide invaluable support in the staging of my PhD art exhibition.

Finally, and during the process of 'writing up', Ian Buchanan (cultural theorist) kindly 'set me straight' on some of the complexities of Deleuzian thought, Ben Anderson (cultural geographer) expanded and challenged my thinking on affect, Nazan Yuksel (teacher) engaged thoughtfully with my short film, Vincent Giles (sound artist) taught me how to expertly 'write with sound', Gordon Chancellor (zoologist) shared specialist knowledge about Charles Darwin's field drawings, Louise Hayes (clinical psychologist) gave me temporary writing space, Stephany Panhuysen (artist) and Michael Ferguson (carpenter) modelled conscientiousness and integrity, Barbara Bolt (artist and academic) was an exceptional mentor, and Christian Edwardes (visual artist/sculptor) shared the PhD writing experience while teaching me things I had not previously known about the neo-avant-garde.

As I have often remarked to Hester, I have been transformed by geography to live a life in relation to a world in which I play but one small part – in contrast to a life constantly at the mercy of internally directed thought. An attunement to the world and the multitude of ways in which we inhabit it as sensing bodies has changed my life. I am convinced that our 'relationscapes' are more important than the singular relation that we so routinely cultivate with our sense of self – a distressing and ultimately unrewarding relationship that occupies so many in the Western world and creates wealth for the professions of psychology and psychiatry in the treatment of the 'worried well'.

July 2016

CONTENTS

1	Introduction	1
2	Process-Oriented Ontologies and the Ethics of Affirmation	5
3	Non-Representational Theory	27
4	Performing Research	43
5	Ekphrastic Geographies	61
6	Interstices of Becoming	91
	References	99
	Index	115

LIST OF FIGURES

Stitching – The fashioning of a felt poppy for the Centenary
of the ANZACs 79
Taking Flight – A moment in a 5rhythms^{TM} dance class when
two dancers leave the ground at the same time 80
Entraining – An act of poetic permaculture where
a human hand winds a banana passion fruit plant around an upright
support 81
Paints – An example of object-oriented photography in which inanimate
materials become portraiture 82
Trace – An example of durational photography where the movement
of a dancer's arm and hair blur to create an image without subject or object 83
River of Fire – One of several photographs, taken during an event
of 'fire-setting' in a storm water drain that went into producing
a stop-frame animation 84
Tricksters – Emerging from underground spaces in unexpected places 85
Tools – A Super 8 camera, an environmental audio-recorder, and
a manual typewriter 86

xiii

CHAPTER 1

Introduction

Abstract This chapter introduces the central proposition of the book – that therapeutic change and transformation are geographical in nature. A brief outline of the book and its contents follows, before turning briefly to the process of 'thinking through practice'.

Keywords Therapeutic space · Ethico-aesthetic paradigm · Post-phenomenology · Transversal thought · The non-representational

This book is about the production of therapeutic space. It considers the ways in which art making, in particular, opens up spaces for the reworking of subjectivities. Rather than conceiving of the subject as 'fixed', this book asserts that the human subject is a 'work in progress'. Furthermore, change and transformation are not outcomes but 'accidents of becoming'. When we allow our 'selves' to get lost in the chaotic potential of the world, we confront the potential for transformation and change (McCormack 2014). Ethico-aesthetic activity produced by sensing bodies dissolves the boundaries between human and non-human, living and non-living in ways that enable us – as human counterparts in a wider geography – to experience 'being singular plural' (Nancy 2000). As Nigel Thrift (2008a) cites: "[r]ather than have to think, always and endlessly, what else there could be, we sometimes seem to connect with a layer in our existence that simply wants the things of the world close to our skin" (Gumbrecht 2004, p. 106).

© The Author(s) 2017
C.P. Boyd, *Non-Representational Geographies of Therapeutic Art Making*, DOI 10.1007/978-3-319-46286-8_1

2 NON-REPRESENTATIONAL GEOGRAPHIES OF THERAPEUTIC ART MAKING

This way of conceptualising the 'therapeutic' as transformative is inspired by the affective turn in the social sciences and humanities – a movement in response to, and alongside, developments in post-phenomenological thought, primarily arising out of France. A radical reformulation of the human subject has taken place within this movement, a formulation only made possible by freeing the human subject from the dictums of science and medicine. For this reason alone, I want to avoid constructions of therapy that arise from psychotherapeutic models of the self. At the same time, however, I need to acknowledge that much of the work of psychotherapy's 'third wave' has been to encourage 'patients' to develop a finer attunement to the world (through the practice of mindfulness) and to foster a cognitive understanding of self as context (see Hayes et al. 2010). While these developments in psychotherapy have led to 'better outcomes' for many, they are constrained by linguistic modes of expression and representational forms of thinking; bringing into question the operations and consequences of inwardly focused psychotherapies and their potential to 're-territorialise' pained subjectivity and human suffering. Instead, in this book, I want to regard therapy as 'thought in action', as 'coming alive in a world of texture', as the development of an attunement to the non-representational, and as the 'performance of one's own subjectivity' (see Manning and Massumi 2014; McCormack 2014; O'Sullivan 2012). In this way, the book has the power to expand current thinking on what constitutes therapy.

A focus on therapeutic space is not to deny that transformative therapeutics operate at the level of the psyche (Collins 2014). In terms of attention, however, it does suspend the psychological in order to foreground the spatial and the material. The case for expressive arts as a catalyst for psychological change is almost non-debatable (Knill et al. 2005). However, exclusively subject-centred understandings of therapeutic art making ignore a whole host of 'other', non-human contributors. In backgrounding the psychological, things like *material* agency, *affect* and the immaterial, *bodily* affordances and rhythms, and the human sensorium come to the fore.

Non-representational theory starts at the body and focuses outwards to affirm relation, regarding the body as a "dynamic-affective, expressive entity" (McCormack 2014, p. 95). Thus, transformative therapeutics considers 'what the body can do', in a similar vein to process-oriented philosophers from Spinoza to Whitehead to Deleuze. It was Félix Guattari, in his solo work *Chaosmosis*, who declared that psychoanalysis should get a grip on life, arguing that language held sovereignty over pragmatics thereby imposing limits on what therapy might achieve (Genosko 2002). For him, basic self-experiences make up the human subject and so therapy must consist of activity that extends us into new, 'fertile' territories.

In order to present a coherent argument in relation to the non-representational geographies of therapeutic art making, this book commences by delving into three distinct, yet overlapping, bodies of literature. The first is process-oriented philosophy, the second is affirmative ethics, and the third is non-representational theory as it emerged from contemporary cultural geography. An understanding of all three areas is necessary to fully justify the fieldwork that was undertaken. These theories not only guide the empirical work but are also enacted by it. The propositions that arise from the work are minor extensions of these domains of thought.

Non-representational theory focuses on 'doings' and is, therefore, interested in practice and performance (Vannini 2015). In terms of research methodology then, non-representational theory necessitates a turn to creative praxis (Thrift 2008a). However, practice as a mode of inquiry already has an established history in the creative arts. Thanks to the concerted efforts of arts academics, performative research methods have now gained acceptance within the academy (Bolt 2010; Haseman 2006; Smith and Dean 2009). Although several geographers have embraced and employed creative methods in their research (e.g., Lorimer and Parr 2014) these tend not to be explicit demonstrations of practice-based knowledge but, rather, an attempt to creatively experiment with different modes of presentation.

Schroeder (2015) argues for the term *practice research* to emphasise that when an artistic researcher employs practice-based methods, artistic practice is at the forefront of the inquiry. 'Practice as research' is a term gaining currency for similar reasons (Nelson 2013). In this book, I instead use the term 'practice-led' in relation to my own research to indicate that as an artist-geographer I am not only led by artistic practice, but I am also led by geography. As a geographer informed by non-representational theory, I cycle through an iterative process of thinking and sensing (see Dewsbury 2009a) which then informs my creative work and how I choose to present it. The creative work itself generates new thought, which then informs my writing.

Working from experience to discourse is a transversal process, and translating practice-based findings into written forms requires a particular mode of thinking. In this regard, the empirical chapter (Chap. 5) employs techniques of 'transversal thought'. As Genosko (2002) describes (after Schrag), transversal thought unfolds across three praxes: *evaluative critique, engaged articulation*, and *incursive disclosure*. 'Evaluative critique' requires discernment – a style of thought that involves separating, sorting out, distinguishing, contrasting, weighting, and assessing (Van Huyssteen 1999). While dissensus, agreement, or the creation of new concepts may be the best way forward, in the transversal play of thought one does not automatically come down on the side of one or another. 'Engaged articulation', on the other hand, is a moment where thought connects with discourse to render an account that attributes sense and meaning to it. Schrag (1994) sees meaning as recollective or anticipative, Genosko (2002) as thought unfolding retentionally and protentionally, which "rescues critique from being simply a strategy of negation and deconstruction" (Van Huyssteen 1999, p. 138). 'Incursive disclosure' brings us back to experience – beyond language and textuality – to postulate a referent outside of the isolated subject to the space of the 'real'.

As an autodidactic artist, I had naive experiences of the artistic process coming into this work. As a scholar new to the disciplines of human geography and the creative arts, I have struggled to find a 'voice' that did not echo the derivative styles of expression upon which the sciences rest. Here, I have found inspiration in the considered, authoritative styles of Elizabeth Grosz and Rosi Braidotti whose complex ideas are expressed with compelling simplicity, the evocative and paratactic styles of Erin Manning and Brian Massumi whose sentence fragments dance across the page providing little 'shocks to the new', and Hélène Cixous' notion of *l'écriture feminine* (Klages 2012) which allowed me to embrace and express what I sensed and felt as a practice researcher.

It is my wish that this book and its various insights will be of benefit to those in the early stages of embarking on new work. And so, this book is for the artistic researchers, the cultural geographers, the social scientists, the psychotherapists, the educationalists, and the independent scholars for whom 'thinking through practice' holds promise.

CHAPTER 2

Process-Oriented Ontologies and the Ethics of Affirmation

Abstract The philosophical underpinnings of the empirical work are described in this chapter in a straightforward manner that makes these complex thinkers more accessible to practice-based researchers. The chapter progresses by philosopher to include contemporary perspectives on process-relational philosophy, post-phenomenology, speculative realism, vital materialisms, and affirmative ethics.

Keywords Process-relational thought · Post-phenomenology · Speculative realism · New materialisms · Affirmative ethics

The philosophies that inform this book also underpin much of the theoretical work produced by cultural geographers interested in affect, performance, and the non-representational (e.g., Dewsbury 2003; McCormack 2003; Thrift 2008a). Collectively, non-representational theorists regard the world, with all its actors and actants, as continually in the process of becoming. As human subjects, the world's unfolding is at the edge of our awareness, occurring at precognitive level – although we, as human subjects, are wholly bound in it. Processes of individuation are intensive. A sea of infinite potential presupposes the present. All entities have the capacity to affect and be affected and enter into relation with each other across a range of spatio-temporal scales. While there may be several ways to organise the ideas that follow – by concept or theme, for example – I present them according to philosopher to maintain what is a discernable lineage in

© The Author(s) 2017   5
C.P. Boyd, *Non-Representational Geographies of Therapeutic Art Making*, DOI 10.1007/978-3-319-46286-8_2

6 NON-REPRESENTATIONAL GEOGRAPHIES OF THERAPEUTIC ART MAKING

the development of thought over time. Primarily, however, I wanted to present these philosophies in a way that transmits the sense of discovery I felt in encountering them. Rather than making oblique references to this material throughout the book, I want to begin by making my own understandings of this material explicit.

ALFRED NORTH WHITEHEAD

Isabelle Stengers, perhaps the foremost Whiteheadian scholar of our time, asserted that "[m]ore than any other philosopher, Whitehead was permeated by a vertiginous distance between the possibilities of the universe and our human abilities to apprehend them" (Stengers 2011, pp. 9–10). Steven Shaviro (2012) also asked what if Alfred North Whitehead was to replace Heidegger as the forerunner of postmodern thought – rather than a concern with being and existence, we might instead ask, "Why is there always something new?"

Recognising that the world is organic (process-based) rather than material (substance-based) is at the heart of Whitehead's speculative philosophy. Process thought regards actuality as a composition of atomic or momentary events, which Whitehead called *actual entities* or *actual occasions* (Whitehead 1978). The enduring objects that humans perceive with their senses are merely strings (or 'societies') of actual occasions, each flowing into the next so they appear to be continuous. This component of *extension* in Whitehead is also a feature of the *event* for Deleuze (Robinson 2010). Events extend over each other in an infinite relation that gives us the illusion of continuity. It is this extension that provides us with our sense of reality.

The ongoing creation of the 'new' for Whitehead is made possible by *prehension*. Prehension is "a non-cognitive *feeling* that guides how the occasion shapes itself from the data of the past and the potentialities of the future" (Robinson 2010, p. 124). Deleuze similarly argued that "[e]verything prehends its antecedents and its concomitants and, by degrees, prehends a world" (Deleuze 1993, p. 78). New entities become present by prehending other entities. Actual entities become themselves as they *concresce* and thereby create all that exists in an evolutionary process that is open rather than predetermined (Marstaller 2009). This describes the creative, ongoing rhythm of life – driven by 'feeling' – that takes place outside of the realm of human consciousness. Our conscious understanding of this physical energy is, according to Whitehead, "an abstraction from the complex energy, emotional and purposeful, inherent

2 PROCESS-ORIENTED ONTOLOGIES AND THE ETHICS OF AFFIRMATION 7

in the subjective form of the final synthesis in which each occasion completes itself" (1933, p. 239).

Whitehead's process-relational philosophy posits a complex world of interlocking experiences – experience that arises from the interaction between subjects and objects (Frisina 2002). Unlike traditional subject–object distinctions, however, Whitehead regards the subject as emerging from its relation with the object, *which itself the subject constitutes*. This understanding of experience rejects the substance-based philosophy that dominated during Whitehead's time. Neither subject nor object are permanent but always reconstitute one another as the subject grasps at the past in order to construct an indeterminate present. Consciousness, rather than being regarded as an independent actuality, is a function of bodily events (Ford 1984).

For Whitehead, there are two kinds of perception: perception in the mode of *causal efficacy* and perception as *presentational immediacy* (Mesle 2008). Presentational immediacy is sense experience. Causal efficacy, however, is the primary mode of perception – our consciousness of the world as constituted by its past. Although we consciously perceive the world in this way, this form of perception is characterised by its vagueness. Presentational immediacy, on the other hand – although considered by Whitehead to be a secondary form of perception – is vivid, lively, and messy. Whereas perception in the mode of causal efficacy is embodied (i.e., we act in relation to the world and perceive that our bodily actions have consequences), in the mode of presentational immediacy we perceive ourselves as being present in another entity: as Whitehead (1978) states, "[w]e find ourselves in a buzzing world amid a democracy of fellow creatures" (p. 50).

Whitehead's 'Ultimate' is creativity – it affirms all that exists and all that happens (Meyer 2005; Stengers 2011). Creativity is activity without purpose or intention and is the principle of novelty. 'Creative advance into novelty' is always happening (Shaviro 2012). Everything with which we deal at any moment in time is an accident of creativity. As Whitehead suggests:

the notion of 'passing on' is more fundamental than that of a private individual fact. In the abstract language here adopted for metaphysical statement, 'passing on' becomes 'creativity', in the dictionary sense of the verb *creare*, 'to bring forth, beget, produce'. Thus, according to [this principle], no entity can be divorced from the notion of creativity. (1978, pp. 212–213)

8 NON-REPRESENTATIONAL GEOGRAPHIES OF THERAPEUTIC ART MAKING

This does not mean that entities are free from the influence of the past. Whitehead describes the past as 'stubborn fact', which cannot be changed and needs to be dealt with in the present (Hosinski 1993). In becoming, there is always something new, but there is always something lost as well, because no temporal occasion can fully prehend its past. As Whitehead (1978) explains, "[o]bjectification requires elimination. The present fact has not the past fact with it in any fully immediacy ... it is an empirical fact that process entails loss" (1978, p. 340).

MAURICE MERLEAU-PONTY

Whitehead's thought provides a particular understanding of the world in which its becomings are at the forefront of experience. We, as human subjects, have agency not as individuals but in dynamic relation with other actors that transform our subjectivity in every, single moment. But what does this mean for the 'sensing body'? Merleau-Ponty's *Phenomenology of Perception* is a philosophy that brings sense perception and space together, which is useful in the light of post-structuralist understandings of what 'the body can do'. Although Merleau-Ponty's thought has been described as an existentialist philosophy (Langer 1989), there are certain affinities between Merleau-Ponty's thought and the post-structuralist critique of experience (see Stoller 2005). Some scholars have gone so far as to assert that his work signalled the end of phenomenology (see Lawlor 2003). Rather than asserting that experience is the foundation of all knowledge, Merleau-Ponty's explicitly problematises the body and the *openness* of experience. Throughout his writings, he defended the concept of pre-predicative experience in reference to its 'primordial', 'pre-conscious', and 'non-thetic' character. Regarding the spatiality of the body, Merleau-Ponty argued that every sensation could be considered as part of a *sensory field*. Sensory fields are spatial in that all sensory objects must occupy space. Every object perceived by a subject belongs to a field of other objects that are not perceived. Furthermore, it is our motility that alerts us to the spatiality of our bodies. As Merleau-Ponty (1962) puts it, "[s]pace is not the setting (real or logical) in which things are arranged, but the means whereby the position of things becomes possible" (p. 288).

For Merleau-Ponty the only way to know our selves is in relation to the world, which is the natural setting for all our thoughts: "[n]othing determines me from outside, not because nothing acts upon me, but, on the contrary, because I am from the start outside myself and open to the world" (1962, p. 530). As Stoller (2005) explains, "[b]y paying attention

2 PROCESS-ORIENTED ONTOLOGIES AND THE ETHICS OF AFFIRMATION   9

to one thing over another within my field of experience, I take on a constitutive role in a process of interpretation in relation to the field of experience" (p. 717). In other words, it is not possible for us to back form our subjectivities by cognitively reflecting on the processes that formed them, as this cognitive activity is always secondary to a pre-reflexive experience of being.

The same might be said for our relationship with other selves in the world, which is described by Merleau-Ponty as 'transcendental'. Transcendental subjectivity reveals itself through interactions with the world and others and is, therefore, a kind of *intersubjectivity*. As such, human subjects are not 'objects' related to 'other objects' in the world but form part of a field of existence. Thus, 'the social' is neither objective nor separable from such field for the purposes of thought. This idea contains an explicit critique of scientism that Merleau-Ponty (1964) framed in the following way:

> Scientific thinking, a thinking which looks on from above, and thinks of the object-in-general, must return to the 'there is' which underlies it; to the site, the should of the sensible and opened world such as it is in our life and for our body ... that actual body I call mine ... Further, associated bodies must be brought forward along with my body. (p. 160)

What then is 'the body'? For Merleau-Ponty, the body is many things. It is a mass of chemical components in interaction, a living organism in a biological milieu, a social subject in a group, and an ego – an impalpable 'thing' composed by habit. Finding inspiration from Gestalt psychology, Merleau-Ponty regarded the body as the 'acquired dialectical ground' on which all higher formations are established through the dynamics of embodiment and habituation. Thus, embodied existence is an extension of the body's practical capacity to act. As Russon (1994) puts it, the body is "the point where I touch the world, where I intervene, and equally, where the world touches me" (p. 295).

In giving primacy to perception, Merleau-Ponty contended that both empiricism and intellectualism fail to appreciate the vitality of the performative human act (see Carman 2008). In the case of empiricism, which regards the body's organs as passive receivers of sense data or qualia, the distinction between the object of experience and our experience of it is collapsed, such that what we perceive is always considered as being apart from our bodies. In contrast, Merleau-Ponty (1962) argued that "we make perception out of the things perceived" (p. 5). If we were not first associated with the objects of our perception, we would not be capable of perceiving them. However, perception is neither a pure act of understanding as in the case of intellectualism. Our understandings are always situated. Pure sensation, in ordinary experience, is a phenomenological field to which we 'give ourselves over' without the need to possess or judge it as truth. As Merleau-Ponty explains:

> In the first case consciousness is too poor, in the second too rich for any phenomenon to appeal compellingly to it. Empiricism cannot see that we need to know what we are looking for, otherwise we would not be looking for it, and intellectualism fails to see that we need to be ignorant of what we are looking for, or equally again we should not be searching. (1962, p. 28)

In terms of method, an embodied approach demands that analytical reflection and scientism be set aside. As Merleau-Ponty (1962) argued, it is only in doing so that it is possible to "rediscover, as anterior to the ideas of subject and object, the fact of my subjectivity and the nascent object, that primordial layer at which both things and ideas come into being" (p. 219). This notion of embodied perception and open receptivity to the world is of great relevance to this book and the way in which practice-based researchers understand the production of art through a 'knowing body' (see Hardy and Danvers 2006).

GILLES DELEUZE AND FÉLIX GUATTARI

Where the 'Ultimate' for Whitehead is creativity, the 'Ultimate' for Deleuze is life itself – there is nothing higher. This is what makes his ontology an affirmative one: life is immanence and desire its constitutive force. Notwithstanding his thoughts on other aspects of metaphysics, Deleuze's individual work and his collaborations with Félix Guattari are profoundly ontological. This is perhaps why his work resonates so strongly with the creative arts.

Scholars can, and do, devote entire careers to the study of Deleuze's thought and yet his writings, as Massumi (1996) asserts, are "intentionally designed to defy summary" (p. 395). There is, therefore, an inherent danger in reducing his thought to a few isolated concepts in the manner that I am about to do. I am encouraged, however, by Deleuze's own ideas about philosophy as generative, even in failure. For Deleuze and Guattari, philosophy, science, logic, and art are all

2 PROCESS-ORIENTED ONTOLOGIES AND THE ETHICS OF AFFIRMATION 11

tools for confronting the world's 'chaos' (Deleuze and Guattari 1994). Putting extraordinary words to ordinary use was also something that Deleuze encouraged (Deleuze and Parnet 1987). In this vein, I will present only four aspects of Deleuzian ontology in this section; they are (1) the actual and the virtual, (2) desiring-production, (3) multiplicity and becoming, and (4) events and singularities, as they are the most pertinent to his metaphysics.

Put simply, the 'actual' is the world as we perceive it in concrete terms, whereas the 'virtual' is the world's infinite potential (i.e., pure multiplicity). The actual and the virtual are not, however, independent of one another, because the actual is in the virtual and the virtual is in the actual (Massumi 2002). As such, the actual and the virtual are mutually presupposed. Actuality unfolds from potentiality, making it possible to intuit the richer potentiality from which the actual emerges (Colebrook 2005). In what is a common misconception, the 'real' is not an actualisation of the virtual – they are both 'real'. It is at the 'seeping edge', however, where the virtual leaks into the actual, that transformation occurs. As Massumi (2002) argues:

> Concepts of the virtual in itself are important only to the extent to which they contribute to a pragmatic understanding of emergence, to the extent to which they enable triggers of change (induce the new). It is the edge of the virtual, where it leaks into actual, that counts. For the seeping edge is where potential, actually, is found. (p. 43)

The actual is not static but is constantly reconfigured through acts of becoming. Therefore, actualisation is a process. For a virtual object to be actualised "is to create divergent lines which correspond to – without resembling – a virtual multiplicity" (Deleuze 1994, p. 212). This process occurs in zones of intensity, which are sites of productive difference (DeLanda 2005). In a reversal of Freudian psychoanalysis, desiring-production works with what is already present in the world rather than being born of unconscious need. It is autonomous, self-constituting, and creative, along the lines of Nietzsche's 'will to power' (Smith and Protevi 2013). Desiring-production is not, however, anthropocentric. What it produces is 'real' and, thus, desire itself is 'actual' (Buchanan 2013).

For Deleuze, multiplicity and becoming are one in the same. This is because multiplicities are always crossing over one another and transforming each other (Deleuze and Guattari 1987). Although composed of several dimensions, a multiplicity is not divisible, because it cannot gain or lose any of its dimensions without changing. In sympathy with Whitehead's process-relational philosophy, being is always secondary to becoming, which is the *a priori* ontological category. As argued in *A Thousand Plateaus*: *"each multiplicity is already composed of heterogeneous terms in symbiosis... a multiplicity is continually transforming itself into a string of other multiplicities according to its thresholds and doors"* (emphasis in the original, Deleuze and Guattari 1987, p. 249).

Deleuzian notions of becoming regard subjectivity as always in motion, yet it is the earth that generates the difference that is the source of these becomings: "[t]he self is only a threshold, a door, a becoming between two multiplicities" (Deleuze and Guattari 1987, p. 249). This notion is not, however, against selfhood. It means that 'being' is univocal and identity a *haecceity*. We have a 'thisness' and a 'hereness and nowness' in which our individuality is expressed (Uhlmann 1996). Duration is thus implicated in becoming in a manner so deftly put by Elizabeth Grosz (2005):

> Duration is the 'field' in which difference lives and plays itself out. Duration is that which undoes as well as what makes: to the extent that duration entails an open future, it involves the fracturing and opening up of the past and the present to what is virtual in them, to what in them differs from the actual, to what in them can bring forth the new. This unbecoming is the very motor of becoming, making the past and present not given but fundamentally ever-altering, virtual. (pp. 4–5)

The *event* is a vital element in Deleuze's conceptualisation of the 'real' as temporal. The event in Deleuzian ontology has its own logics, which Deleuze derived from several sources including Whitehead, the 'Stoics', and Leibniz (Robinson 2010). Most importantly, however, events never reproduce themselves; they always invent something new. Another condition of events is their extension. In extension, the event is, in of itself, an 'imbrication'... and unlimited in that it is infinitely divisible (Bowden 2011). The event is also effectuated. As Lawlor (2012) states, "[w]hat makes the event new is that it is caused, accidentally or by chance" (p. 116). Ultimately, events counter-effectuate and feed back into the virtual in a reversal of intensity thereby contemporaneously creating difference (Viveiros de Castro 2012).

2 PROCESS-ORIENTED ONTOLOGIES AND THE ETHICS OF AFFIRMATION 13

Within the constant flow of events are moments or points of tension within matter or things that are utterly unique. Deleuze refers to this component of the event as a *singularity*. In his words "[s]ingularities are turning points and points of inflection; bottlenecks, knots, foyers, and centers; points of fusion and condensation, and boiling; points of tears and joy, sickness and health, hope and anxiety, 'sensitive' points" (Deleuze 1990, p. 63). Within singularities are all the variations within the field, or what Massumi (1996) refers to as a 'co-presencing' of potential. This component of the event is intension rather than extension. Processes of individuation take place in these moments, appearing only by degrees (Duffy 2012). As such, Deleuzian ontology presents the 'real' as dynamic, open-ended, never lacking and always unfolding. Insomuch as it is profoundly ontological, Deleuze's work is also a 'geophilosophy'. As human subjects, we are always becoming in relation, not as individual actors but as 'a mixture of bodies' – mutually affecting one another in our habitation of the earth.

JEAN-LUC MARION, JEAN-LUC NANCY, AND CATHERINE MALABOU

Referred to by some researchers as post-phenomenology (e.g., Ash and Simpson 2014; Simpson 2009), the new generation of French philosophers, although inspired by phenomenologists, share a rejection of the linguistic paradigm, possess a renewed interest in the concrete and the material, and engage in a radical re-framing of the human subject (James 2012). While the term 'new French philosophy' extends to the political philosophies of Jacques Rancière, François Laruelle, and Bernard Stiegler, the focus in this chapter continues to entertain questions of ontology and subjectivity as they potentially relate to the micro-politics of art making in therapeutic spaces. As such, Jean-Luc's Marion's thought on the appearance and givenness of phenomena; Jean-Luc Nancy's thinking on the post-phenomenological subject; and Catherine Malabou's 'plastic reading' of Heidegger are foregrounded in this section.

As a post-phenomenologist, Jean-Luc Marion argued that phenomena are given on their own terms and not limited by the subject that perceives them. The appearing of phenomena is completely unconditional and free from any external circumstances. The subject passively 'receives' a phenomenon as it

14 NON-REPRESENTATIONAL GEOGRAPHIES OF THERAPEUTIC ART MAKING

appears, not as a sovereign ego but as an *adonné* (or one who becomes temporally engaged). The subject is thus transformed by the receiving (Mackinlay 2010). The giving of a phenomenon to a subject that receives it does not 'found or ground anything': the phenomenon simply makes itself manifest in ways that are utterly irreducible and unconstrained. As Marion states, "being never intervenes in order to permit the absolute givenness in which it plays not the slightest role" (Marion 1998, p. 43).

Although Marion regards all phenomena as given, his philosophy introduces a new category of phenomena – the *saturated*. Saturated phenomena are characterised by "so much intuition that they exceed any concepts or limiting horizons that a constituting subject might attempt to impose on them" (Mackinlay 2010, p. 11). Compared to 'common' phenomena, saturated phenomena cannot be aimed at – they are unexpected, unpredictable, and without intentional directedness. Furthermore, saturated phenomena are not dependent upon the intensity with which they appear but upon the way in which they *exceed* any particular horizon; they are unavailable, un-manageable, non-(re)producible, unmasterable (Marion 2004).

To the human subject, saturated phenomena appear in four modalities – the event, the idol, the flesh, and the icon (James 2012). Historical events that qualify as saturated phenomena are those whose impact exceeds the intentional directedness or expectations of the populations they affect. The election of Adolf Hitler to the German parliament in 1933 is one example. For the idol, Marion makes specific reference to works of art, particularly paintings. He argues that a painting always gives the subject a sensory experience that exceeds any interpretation or classification to which it might otherwise be assigned. Moreover, the invisible offered by a painting can only appear if it is received by one who has the aptitude to see it – one who remains open to its 'appearing'. As Marion puts it, "[t]he painting is still seen in a fitting way as long as a gaze exposes itself to it as to an event that arises anew – it remains seen as long as one tolerates the fact that it happens as an event" (Marion 2002, p. 48).

In sympathy with the work of Merleau-Ponty, the third modality of saturated phenomena is flesh. For Marion, the experiences of the flesh, such as pain or pleasure, are *auto-affections* – that is, they occur prior to any intentional directedness or consciousness. Furthermore, the flesh gives the self to itself insomuch as it reveals itself as a phenomenon that cannot be signified. The fourth and final modality of saturated phenomena is the icon. Marion describes the icon as "that which offers nothing to the gaze

2 PROCESS-ORIENTED ONTOLOGIES AND THE ETHICS OF AFFIRMATION   15

and which, inaccessible to the gaze of a spectator, nevertheless imposes its own gaze upon the spectator" (James 2012, p. 35). In accordance with Levinas, one example of this modality is the 'irregardability' of the face. The face of another person does not simply self-manifest but is envisaged by the receiver with a necessary degree of openness. The face is not simply gazed upon but gazes back in an inversion of intentionality (Mackinlay 2010).

While Jean-Luc Marion's thought emphasises the character and appearance of phenomena, Jean-Luc Nancy engages more fully with post-phenomenological postulates of the subject as decentred. In *Being Singular Plural*, Nancy argues that nothing of the world can be sensed in isolation. Sense is always given to an 'us' in a way that can only ever be shared: "[e]xistence *is with*: otherwise nothing exists" (emphasis in the original, Nancy 2000, p. 4). Even internally directed thought, which may be perceived as solely possessed by me, is a communication between me and myself and so is yet another example of 'being with'.

Nancy's account of the 'singular plural' is fundamentally spatial as everything passes between an 'us'. This does not mean, however, that everything passes from one to another or is even connected to one or the other. For Nancy, 'being with' is an interlacing: *contiguity* not continuity and not connection. Even the experience of proximity or closeness emphasises the distance that it opens up – the 'between' is a stretching out, or spacing, of meaning. Being is given to us as 'meaning in circulation', and we *are* that circulation. As Nancy (2000) explains:

> Being cannot be anything but being-with-one-another circulating in the with and as the with of this singularly plural coexistence … But this circulation goes in all directions at once, in all directions of all the space-times [*les espace-temps*] opened by presence to presence: all things, all beings, all entities, everything past and future, alive, dead, inanimate, stones, plants, nails, gods – and "humans". (p. 3)

In *The Birth to Presence*, Nancy's thinking is initially offered in direct contrast to representational thought, which he argues is limited by its own form such that nothing new can be born from it. To be 'born', for Nancy, is to be 'formless'– to be 'in the midst of taking place', without beginning or end: " '[t]o be' is not yet to have been, and already to have been" (Nancy 1993, p. 2). To be born is to be exposed to our existence in every moment of every day. Thought cannot expose this experience to us, because thought forecloses being. Before and after the subject – its consciousness and its 'representational grasp' – there is the coming and going, the back and forth of all there is. The subject is merely thrown into being, or born into presence. As Nancy describes, "[e]xperience is just this, being born to the presence of a sense, a presence itself nascent, and only nascent. Such is the destitution, such the freedom of experience" (1993, p. 4).

Being as a form of exchange is also a feature of Catherine Malabou's 'plastic' reading of Heidegger's *Being and Time*. For Malabou, metaphysics is the history of an exchange between being and beings. Her desire in performing a unique reading of Heidegger's work was to bring to the fore three concepts she believed were radically important to the 'metaphysics of man' but which were constrained by Heidegger's own frame. The three concepts she elaborates in her reading are *Wandeln* (change), *Wandlungen* (transformation), and *Verwandlungen* (metamorphoses), which collectively she refers to as 'the triad of change' (Malabou 2004). Although each of these concepts encapsulates notions of mutation, conversion, or turning-into, they can be considered to operate along two principal axes – a migratory axis and a metamorphic one. This is because "'change' always means at once *change of route and change of form*" (Malabou 2004, p. 19).

Regarding migration, Malabou makes reference to Heidegger's reading of Hölderlin's hymn titled *The Ister*. Here, migration is characterised by a 'strolling about', an 'incessant and directionless change' or 'travelling without destination'. As "Heidegger declares, '[c]hange has here the sense of migrating, going, but at the same time of becoming other' … Change takes shape, then, as a way forward while paths, reciprocally are revealed to be continually changing" (Malabou 2004, p. 20). Change is conceived as 'progress without aim' – taking place through a series of bends or turns where 'advance' is at once a turning back and 'progression' is *wandering* or *meandering*. For Heidegger, however, any real change also involves a change in form (a metamorphosis), which occurs in correlation with migratory change. For Malabou, "the 'transformation of human-ness,' is in effect 'a displacing [of] its site among beings' … a different form at the same time as it is cast as following 'another direction'" (2004, p. 22).

Malabou's more recent writings extend into the realm of contemporary neuroscience (Malabou 2008), the full extent of which will not be discussed here. She does, however, offer some reflections on subjectivation that are pertinent to this book. While firmly believing in the 'self' as a product of a neuronal brain, Malabou upholds Foucault's notion of trans-subjectivation,

2 PROCESS-ORIENTED ONTOLOGIES AND THE ETHICS OF AFFIRMATION 17

suggesting that the concept is thoroughly consistent with her own thoughts on plasticity and change. In conversation with Noëlle Vahanian, Malabou declares:

> [trans-subjectivation] ... consists of a trajectory *within* the self. This trans-subjectivation doesn't mean that you become *different* from what you used to be, nor that you are able to absorb the other's *difference* but that you open a space within yourself between two forms of yourself. That you oppose two forms of yourself within yourself. Foucault writes: "Clear a space around the self and do not let yourself be carried away and distracted by all the sounds, faces, and people around you" ... This transsubjectivation, conceived as a journey within oneself, is a product of a transformation. (Vahanian 2008, p. 5)

Although each makes a unique contribution to post-phenomenological thought, Marion, Nancy, and Malabou all engage with notions of a decentred subject that gesture towards a geography of 'appearing worlds'. Marion does so by presenting an argument for the primacy of phenomena – independent from any subject who may receive them; Nancy articulates the concept of 'being with' such that 'we' are always in relation and in circulation with one another; and Malabou emphasises the mutability of being in ways that implicate processes of change and transformation.

QUENTIN MEILLASSOUX, GRAHAM HARMAN, AND JANE BENNETT

Referred by several names including 'new materialism', 'vital materialism', 'neo-materialism', and 'speculative materialism', a collective interest in the ontological status of objects has recently emerged across a range of academic disciplines, including the creative arts (Barrett and Bolt 2013; Bolt 2007; Bryant et al. 2011; Dieter 2013). Whether part of human and non-human assemblages or beyond human altogether, this renewed focus on objects and their materialities has a myriad of implications, not only for contemporary metaphysics but for ethics and epistemology as well. Although the contributions to this 'new tradition' are varied and diverse (see Dolphijn and van der Tuin 2012), this discussion is confined to two. The first is the speculative materialism of Quentin Meillassoux and the object-oriented ontology of Graham Harman – complementary perspectives on the materialities of 'things' encompassed by the term 'speculative

18 NON-REPRESENTATIONAL GEOGRAPHIES OF THERAPEUTIC ART MAKING

realism'. The second is the vital materialism of Jane Bennett as outlined in her book, *Vibrant Matter*.

In an essay that appeared in the independent journal *Collapse*, Quentin Meillassoux outlines his thoughts on the non-correlation of events and the necessity of contingency. Further expounded in his book *After Finitude*, Meillassoux's argument is that if it is not possible to prove the 'effective necessity' of the connections between events then we should abandon the problem (Hume's problem) in preference for a different ontological approach. According to Meillassoux (2007), this ontology has a double exigency: "that which is given to experience, and the critique of representation" (p. 81). While everything we know comes from experience, 'everything we know' is not all that there is. The world envisaged by Meillassoux is a 'hyperchaos' – where constants change in every single instant for 'no reason whatsoever'. As he puts it:

> New sets of possibilities … irrupt, from nothing, as no external structure contains them as external potentialities before their emergence, we thus make *irruption* ex nihilo *the very concept of a temporality delivered to its pure immanence.* (emphasis in the original, Meillassoux 2007, p. 72)

Meillassoux also argues that this 'metaphysics of chance' forces a rethinking of becoming. If the only law of the universe is the necessity of contingency then becoming is an even more radical process than previously understood by philosophers. Rather than a process imposed on the world by time, time can bring forth 'the new' in ways that are unconstrained by any precedent situation.

Although a great deal of dissent exists among those who identify as speculative realists (see Harman 2013), there are two, related principles that they uphold. The first principle relates to the inner vitality of objects (in of themselves), and the second relates to non-correlationism – the fact that objects exist independently of their relations (Harman 2002; Meillassoux 2009). In an essay published in 2012 as part of an art exhibition, Graham Harman illustrates these points via the analogy of 'the third table' (see Harman 2012). Borrowing from a famous lecture by British astrophysicist Sir Arthur Stanley Eddington, Harman begins his essay by comparing the classical 'two tables' of Eddington's scenario. The 'first table' is an object that we use in everyday life – to eat at, to write on, to set things upon. The 'second table', however, is the one described by physics – a table composed of atoms and their electrons in constant motion.

2 PROCESS-ORIENTED ONTOLOGIES AND THE ETHICS OF AFFIRMATION 19

While Eddington argues the 'real' table is the second one as understood by science, and not the first one as understood by the humanities, Harman argues that neither table is 'real'. Both of Eddington's alternatives reduce the table to only some of its characteristics: in the first instance the table is reduced to a human–object relation, and in the second instance, the table is reduced to its chemical components and their interactions. Neither of these understandings adequately accounts for the entirety of the object. Instead Harman posits a 'third table' – a table that has an *autonomous* reality separate from its usefulness to humans and consisting of emergent properties that cannot be solely inferred from the interactions among its component parts. Interestingly, Harman suggests that the only paradigm capable of apprehending the third table is the creative arts, as it is the only 'culture' that does not seek to reduce the table in any way.

Regarding objects for human use, Harman makes an ontic distinction between *readiness-to-hand* and *present-at-hand* (Harman 2002). Readiness-to-hand refers the ability of objects to completely withdraw from human view into a 'dark subterranean reality' that never becomes present. Even in becoming present-at-hand (i.e., into relation with a human subject), objects still withhold their deepest being as it is never possible for it to be fully revealed through interaction. Meillassoux (2009) puts this in another way. While he accepts that 'the sensible' only exists in a subject's relation to the world, he also suggests that (mathematisable) properties of objects are exempt from this relation.

In accordance with (and beyond) the propositions of Meillassoux and Harman, Jane Bennett argues that non-human forces are active participants in worldly events. She calls these forces 'thing power' (Bennett 2010). 'Thing-power' for Bennett is the fact that things affect knowing bodies in ways that are independent of any sovereign influence. Because materiality is vitally intrinsic to all things whether organic or inorganic, we, as humans, can be thought of as non-human as well – in that we are also vitally material. Consistent with the ideas of Merleau-Ponty, Bennett suggests that the living body extends to the whole sensible world. Prompted by the materialities of our bodies, we are capable of discovering the myriad of ways in which 'objects' are also forces of expression. According to Bennett, "[v]ital materialists will [thus] linger in those moments during which they find themselves fascinated by objects, taking them as clues to the material vitality that they share with them" (2010, p. 17). While Bennett, in the same vein as speculative realists, stresses that 'things' have a 'reality' which is intrinsic to them, she is much more concerned with the extent to which human beings and 'thinghood' overlap to produce political and behavioural ecologies. As Bennett (2010) explains, a materiality is "as much a force as entity, as much energy as matter, as much intensity as extension" (2010, p. 20).

In thinking about the nature of *distributive agency*, Bennett deploys Deleuze and Guattari's notion of the 'assemblage'. In an ecological sense, assemblages are finite groupings of diverse elements that work together to produce effects. The agency of an assemblage is not under the control of any one element: the effects that are generated by them are best considered as 'emergent properties'. While it is possible for members of an assemblage to act with will or intentionality, these 'willed' actions become part of 'the mix', overlapping with the agency of other things which have conflicting degrees of power and efficacy: "[h]ere causality is more emergency than efficient, more fractal than linear ... [rather than] an effect obedient to a determinant, one finds circuits in which effect and cause alternate position and redound on each other" (Bennett 2010, p. 33).

'Assemblage thinking' has radical applications for some of the world's most pressing problems. It also, however, has implications for the mundane and the every day. Fundamentally for Bennett, the primary purpose of vital materialism is to upset the belief that human beings are special. We do not exist outside of our own materiality. Our vitality is distributed along an ontological continuum. Our will and intentionality overlap with the conflicting power of 'things'. The locus of agency is in human–non-human assemblages and not the human 'ego'. Far from disabling, however, an attunement to the intrinsic vitality of objects has the potential to liberate. In Bennett's words:

> We are now in a better position to name that other way to promote human health and happiness: *to raise the status of the materiality of which we are composed*. Each human is a heterogeneous compound of wonderfully vibrant, dangerously vibrant, matter. If matter itself is lively, then not only is the difference between subjects and objects minimized, but the status of the shared materiality of all things is elevated (emphasis in the original). (Bennett 2010, pp. 12–13)

Félix Guattari

Félix Guattari, in his solo works, was primarily concerned with promulgating ethical openness by rethinking the basis of human subjectivity (Guattari 1995). In the context of an ethico-aesthetic paradigm, he envisaged three

2 PROCESS-ORIENTED ONTOLOGIES AND THE ETHICS OF AFFIRMATION 21

ecologies within which creative methods of living and acting might be nurtured and developed (Guattari 1989). These three interlocking ecologies, after Bateson, are environmental, social, and mental – corresponding to the biosphere, social relations, and human subjectivity. Guattari's three ecologies radically decentre social struggles to promote modes of becoming that are *transversal*. According to Guattari (1989) we must learn to think transversally: to do so is to respect difference, affirm life, and resist hegemony. Ecology is not a 'love of environment' but the whole of subjectivity and capitalistic power formations (Guattari 2013). Ecophosy (or thinking ecologically) is a method of being with the purpose of creating a sustainable and equitable form of human existence. Ultimately, Guattari's ethico-aesthetic paradigm is a therapeutic ethos. It is *contra* to psychoanalytic and symbolic notions of desire as individual and interior (constituted by lack) and instead sees desire as a positive force that flows in and through 'the social'. As Guattari (1989) asserts:

> To bring into being worlds other than those of pure abstract information; to engender universes of reference and existential territories in which singularity and finitude are embraced by the multivalent logic of mental ecologies and the social-ecological group … to face up to a dizzying confrontation with the cosmos in order to make it in some way liveable; these are, in short, the intertwining paths of the triple ecological vision to which we should now turn all attention. (p. 147)

For Guattari, subjectivity always remains 'unmerged', coexisting, and interacting (Genosko 2002). It is plural and polyphonic and takes place in confrontation with new materials of expression. It is, therefore, not a subjectivity but 'subjectivation' – an *autopoiēsis*, a processual creativity, the 'schizo' unconscious turned towards praxis. According to Guattari (1995), we constantly move between de-territorialisation (freeing ourselves from the restrictions and boundaries of controlled, striated spaces) and re-territorialisation (repositioning ourselves within striated spaces). In contrast, smooth spaces are liminal, open, and dynamic spaces that allow for creativity to take place more easily through unpredictable lines of flight. Lines of flight may be destructive or productive (or both) as they may either enable or diminish affective capacities. Ethico-aesthetic practices, however, operate transversally – vertically and horizontally. "Transversal movements drive subjectivities in directions alternative to those aligned with prescribed subjective territories" (Reynolds 2009, p. 2). Such moments are best understood as a 'praxic opening' to the virtual potential that the world holds for subjectivation (Genosko 2002). Or, as Massumi (1995) calls it, an 'affective escape' – the perception of one's own vitality and changeability.

It was Guattari's vision that the human and social sciences shift from a scientific paradigm to an ethico-aesthetic one – away from psychoanalysis and 'back to life'. His method, developed with psychiatric patients at the La Borde clinic in France, implemented pragmatic interventions that encouraged the construction of new subjectivities by opening up new fields of virtuality (Guattari 1995). Subjectivities were re-singularised within a climate of activity, based on shared responsibility, which fostered collective subjectivation via multiple exchanges between individual–group–machine. Components of the patient's environment – the architecture, the clinic's economy, the transversal relationships with staff – allowed patients to "[take] advantage of all occasions opening onto the outside world; a processual exploitation of event-centred 'singularities' [where] everything can contribute to the creation of an authentic relation with the other" (Guattari 1995, p. 7). Subjectivity was seen not as the purvey of the individual but as a co-mingling of relations – assemblages of enunciation (or expression) that create universes of value. By learning to sense things differently, the patients at La Borde experimented with new means of expression and novel approaches to living; as Genosko (2002) suggests "even the simplest idea that subjectivity is not interiority but the product of diverse *existential dispositions* is liberating in therapeutic contexts" (emphasis added, p. 104). Pragmatic approaches to therapy, such as those employed at La Borde, foreground what it is possible to know through affective contamination. New ways of thinking and behaving are not developed through application but by participation in the world.

Guattari's approach to therapy at La Borde has much in common with contemporary art practices, including socially-engaged art. Practices such as these engage directly with the 'texture of living' to transversally affect and transform social dynamics in acts of political resistance or dissent (Thompson 2012; Sullivan 2006; O'Sullivan and Stahl 2006; Zepke 2011). Guattari, however, did not see this as just the work of artists (O'Sullivan 2010). Ethico-aesthetics is a 'will to art' – "a subjective creativity which traverses the generations" (Guattari 1995, p. 91). Art is a mode of production. What it produces is affects. Although, art making is not the limit of Guattari's aesthetic paradigm, it holds a "privileged role in the production of subjectivity" (O'Sullivan 2012, p. 92). As O'Sullivan (2012) explains, the making of art is a form of 'self-overcoming' which allows an 'infolding' of the subject back into him or herself in an act of self-care which "constitutes a freedom of sorts from subjection" (p. 95). This act also involves a folding in of the outside (or the infinite) in a gesture of self-mastery and self-organisation.

Guattari sheds further light on the processes of subjectivation, or 'the energetics of existence', in his book *Schizoanalytic Cartographies*. Within a cartography of assemblages, Guattari elaborates four interrelated 'functors' in diagrammatic form (see Watson 2009, for elucidation). According to Guattari, transformation involves all four domains. The four 'functors', after Aristotle, are flows (F) of matter (*causa materialis*); machinic phyla (Φ) including abstract machines (*causa formalis*); existential territories (T) including 'selfhood' (*causa efficiens*); and universes (U) of value (*causa finalis*). Flows refer to the smooth and non-linear way in which the world presents itself in space–time as a 'form of fluctuation' or a 'material continuum'. Machinic phyla, in contrast, are formed out of the articulation of *substantial* and *expressive de-territorialisations* that bring order to chaos in the form of devices, rules, and regulations. These dimensions cannot, however, achieve existential consistency without involving territories and universes of value. Existential territories comprise multiple, dominant, or minor *refrains* that singularise and re-singularise subjectivities, while universes of value represent non-discursive fields of reference that are not yet real or actualised. Assemblages of enunciation 'smooth' machinic phyla in a variety of ways such that the individuated 'subject' (who speaks in the first person) is nothing more than a fluctuating intersection, or the conscious 'terminal' of these diverse components of temporalisation (Guattari 2013, p. 206). Thus, subjectivation within Guattari's diagrammatic thought is always an open-ended and speculative enterprise, best characterised as a kind of 'existential grasping'. As Jellis (2014) notes, "Guattari's method is in keeping with the ethos of many non-representational theories that understand the world as incomplete and inconsistent, necessitating an approach that is animated by a spirit of affirmative experimentation."

ROSI BRAIDOTTI AND LUCE IRIGARAY

As Guattari suggests, the subject is not separate from this world but embedded in it. Subjectivity is not a self-creation but an autopoēsis, an opening to praxis. The subject emerges from the world on which it depends – in relation and always more than one (Manning 2013; Yuksoff 2014).

24 NON-REPRESENTATIONAL GEOGRAPHIES OF THERAPEUTIC ART MAKING

This is the basic position of post-phenomenological and post-structuralist thinkers; that the human cannot be separated from the non-human, and the 'self' is always intersubjective. Rosi Braidotti's term for this concept is the 'nomadic subject' (Braidotti 2006, 2011a). Possessed of a nomadic consciousness, the nomadic subject goes beyond intentionality and iden-tification. Rather than indulging in acts of self-making, an ethical subject emerges from multiple processes of becoming – becoming-animal, becom-ing-world, and, ultimately, becoming-imperceptible. In order to enter into finer processes of becoming one must first 'die to the self'. As she explains:

> Not the least paradox involved in this process is that in order to trigger a process of becoming-imperceptible, quite a transformation needs to take place in what we could call the self. Becoming-imperceptible is the point of fusion between the self and his or her habitat, the cosmos as a whole. It marks the point of evanescence of the self and its replacement by a living nexus of multiple interconnections that empower not the self, but the collective, not identity, but affirmative subjectivity, not consciousness, but affirmative interconnections. It is like a flood gate of creative forces that make it possible to be actually fully inserted into the *hic et nunc* defined as the present unfolding of potentials, but also the enfolding of qualitative shifts within the subject. (p. 261)

Such qualitative shifts involve the transposition of negative affects into positive affects. As Braidotti argues, the ethical subject is one who recog-nises that he or she has the power to depersonalise events and their negative 'charge': "[e]very event contains with it the potential for being overcome and overtaken – its negative charge can be transposed" (Braidotti 2011b, p. 288). What is negative about certain affects and events is not their moral value but their effects: negative affects close off potential; they diminish capacities. For this reason, they "should neither be encouraged, nor should we be rewarded for lingering around them too long" (Braidotti 2011b, p. 288).

For Braidotti, the vitalist notion of *zoe* is important as it emphasises that 'my life is not mine' – it is a 'generative force of becoming'. This view resonates with the philosophy of Merleau-Ponty in which the body can never be considered as separate from its field of experience. David Abram (1996) calls this *perception as participation*. For Abram, 'inanimate' objects are alive in that they can be experienced sensorially. The perceiving body always involves an active interplay with the environment. The world

2 PROCESS-ORIENTED ONTOLOGIES AND THE ETHICS OF AFFIRMATION 25

is always 'disclosing' itself to us in its unfolding: "at the most primordial level of sensuous, bodily experience, we find ourselves in an expressive, gesturing landscape, in a world that *speaks*" (emphasis in the original; Abram 1996, p. 81). Furthermore, this active participation in the world is always unfinished as the 'flux' of participation is ceaseless.

Part of an active participation in the world is a sense of wonder. To wonder is to stop and rest, to look towards the other, to contemplate – sometimes in very 'ordinary' ways (Stewart 2007). According to Irigaray (1993), wonder is first and foremost a will to move. Things must be appealing to the senses in order to be desired, and desire makes us act. Wonder is both active and passive, however. It is a call to witness, and it is the 'ground' – or what Irigaray describes as 'the inner secret of genesis, or creation'. As she asserts:

> Wonder [is] the passion of encounter between the most material and the most metaphysical, of their possible conception and fecundation one by the other. A third dimension. An intermediary. Neither the one nor the other. Which is not to say neutral or neuter. The forgotten ground of our condition between mortal and immortal, men and gods, creatures and creators. In us and among us. (p. 82)

Through the sensing body, we wonder in spite of ourselves. Put another way, wonder de-territorialises us (Bertelson 2013). Bennett (2001) calls this condition of exhilaration, or acute sensory experience, enchantment. Enchantment is "[t]o be simultaneously transfixed in wonder and transported by sense, to be both caught up and carried away...[an] odd combination of somatic effects" (Bennett 2001, p. 5). For Bennett (2001), enchantment is critical for the cultivation of an *aesthetic disposition* – an ethical stance that holds 'brute feeling' and 'sublime Reason' in a delicate balance (see also Tauber 2006). To wonder with the world is to develop an affective model of ethics that does not reduce it to "a narcisstic practice of care of the self" (p. 133). As Guattari's clinical practices demonstrate, new ways of being are created through participation, not prescription or application. Human becoming is, therefore, geographical – an assertion which disrupts traditional notions of self as interior and which is explored further in the empirical work to come.

CHAPTER 3

Non-Representational Theory

Abstract This chapter introduces non-representational theory to an inter-disciplinary audience by unpacking some of its key concepts – movement, joint action, precognition, embodiment, and affect. The chapter ends by considering the ways in which non-representational theory promotes a particular view of 'space' as intensive.

Keywords Non-representational theory · Joint action · Precognition · Corporeality · Affect

The goal of this chapter is to present non-representational theory, as I understand it – as a product of my engagement with it. While I focus exclusively on non-representational theory as it emerged from British social and cultural geography in the 1990s, it is important to acknowledge that non-representational theories traverse several modes of thinking in the social sciences, humanities, and the creative arts – particularly, performance studies. In geography, however, non-representational theory is spatially inflected and, due to this inflection, non-representational geographers think very differently about the human subject. For us, the human subject is distributed across space-time, constantly in the process of entering into, and departing from, temporally unstable relations between a multitude of actors and actants, all of which are doing the same. Furthermore, these events of coming into relation are not causally connected. After Whitehead, the

© The Author(s) 2017   27
C.P. Boyd, *Non-Representational Geographies of Therapeutic Art Making*, DOI 10.1007/978-3-319-46286-8_3

'flow of time' is a fallacy of sorts in that it is made up of a succession of singularities, which can only be 'stored' by representation.

While this way of thinking about the world is enticing, it also opens up a raft of aporias with which students and scholars new to non-representational theory often struggle. I am yet to resolve them for myself but have instead evolved a strategy for keeping them 'in suspension'. Scholars in the creative arts, I suspect, have been cultivating similar strategies for some time. The apparent validity of 'practice as research' and the academy's insistence that research be written down create a similar sort of tension. Essentially, non-representational theory is a philosophical project that is impossible to put fully into practice. As pointed out by J-D Dewsbury, however, whatever is gained by failing still counts as knowledge (Dewsbury 2009a).

A Geography of What Happens

Non-representational theory in geography was 'hatched' by Nigel Thrift as a critical response to human geography's obsession with representation (Thrift 2008a). To appreciate the need for Thrift's response, it is first necessary to understand what representation is and what it does. To this end, Richard Rorty provides a provocative summary in his book *Philosophy and the Mirror of Nature*. He argues that from the seventeenth century onwards, and in an endeavour to elevate itself to the 'queen of sciences', philosophy invented epistemology. Since then, the chief occupation of philosophy has been mental representations and their accuracy. As Rorty (1979) puts it:

> To know is to represent accurately what is outside the mind; so to understand the possibility and nature of knowledge is to understand the way in which the mind is able to construct such representations. Philosophy's central concern is to be a general theory of representation, a theory which will divide culture up into the areas which represent reality well, those which represent it less well, and those which do not represent it at all. (despite their pretence of doing so; p. 3)

Michel Foucault also critically engaged with representational knowledge, but unlike Rorty, asserted that representations are *social facts* (Foucault 1971). They are problematic insomuch as they are linked to a wide range of social and political practices that make up the Western world – a world in which order, truth, and the subject are paramount. Social order, domination and resistance, marginalisation, and inequality have been the concern of social scientists for decades (Rabinow 1986). As such, formal techniques of representation are routinely employed in their discourses. The practice of representation becomes contentious, however, when representations cease to be problematised by those who deploy them.

For Nigel Thrift, the problem with representational thinking has less to do with what it does and more to do with what it leaves out. Representations are oriented towards a world that is already there, whereas non-representational theory is best described as *"the geography of what happens"* (emphasis in the original; Thrift 2008a, p. 2). Non-representational theory embraces uncertainty by affirming life's 'messiness'. It does so not by reinventing epistemology but by theoretically and methodologically foregrounding the processes of life's emergence. The use of 'non' rather than 'more-than' assists in this endeavour by emphasising that which is "undisclosed" (Harrison 2007, p. 174). Non-representational theory is interested in the way that life 'takes place' through movement, intensities, and encounters (Lorimer 2005). It challenges the realm of language and its economy by asserting that there is always more going on than what we can apprehend (Dewsbury 2010). Moreover, non-representational theory is a way of thinking about the world that places humans on equal footing with everything else. As Thrift suggests, the world is "jam-packed with entities" that simultaneously enter into, and out of, relation with one another (2008a, p. 17) – humans are wrapped up in a wider ecology of 'things'.

In positing a geography of what happens, non-representational theory takes movement as its *leitmotif* (see Thrift 2008a) and sees living as a "succession of luminous or mundane instances" (p. 5). All life is based on and in movement. Movement is the 'stuff of life', capturing the joy of living. Matter and movement have no way of expressing what is in becoming, because they are always in excess of language (Dewsbury 2010). It is in "the performances that make us, that the world comes about" (Dewsbury et al. 2002, p. 439). As such, the concept of *on-flow* is central to non-representational styles of thought. Drawing on the work of process-relational philosophers, non-representational theory gives primacy to the world's unfolding. The world is emergent, and we (as human subjects) play but one small role in its actualisation. We live *through* what is happening. While we experience the world as an embodied subject, the body has a particular inability to contain or regulate itself. We are typically overwhelmed by events. As Dewsbury et al. suggest:

First, the world calls us to witness it into being. We are "caught in the fabric of the world" (Merleau-Ponty 1969, p. 256), cast in its materiality, in a

30 NON-REPRESENTATIONAL GEOGRAPHIES OF THERAPEUTIC ART MAKING

world of transubjective modalities of experience, an in-between world of imperatives instigating our activities. (p. 439)

As such, the status of the subject is diminished in non-representational theory. The subject merely emerges from a world in which it is entangled. Thus, non-representational theory is more interested in *subjectivation* than subjectivity. Through practice, *matter as agency* is distributed between object and subject, human and non-human. Practices are understood as working styles that have the appearance of stability over time through the "establishment of corporeal routines and specialized devices, to reproduce themselves" (Thrift 2008a, p. 8). As Anderson and Harrison (2010) assert, "the root of action is to be conceived less in terms of willpower or cognitive deliberation and more via embodied and environmental affordances, dispositions and habits" (p. 7).

Habit presents a peculiar paradox for non-representational theory due to its apparent "dual logic of continuity and change" (Bissell 2012). Drawing on Félix Ravaisson's 1834 work *On Habit*, non-representational geographers have argued that a passive and active sense resides in our bodies such that we are simultaneously *adapted* and *adaptive* (Dewsbury 2012). For Ravaisson (2008), habits form a kind of 'background ecology' against which spontaneous action takes place, producing an open-ended temporality (see Grosz 2013). In this way, the force of habit anticipates spontaneity by preparing the body for action. Bissell (2012) puts the notion of habit to work in thinking through obduracy and the ways in which the body sometimes struggles to move. Habit, for Bissell, tends towards volatility in order that we might participate in "the more unstable, precarious and heterogeneous modulations of contemporary life" (2012, n.p.). In terms of movement, this conceptualisation of habit enables non-representational geographers to conceive of 'stillness' as a form of mobility – as part of the habitual rhythm of the everyday (Bissell and Fuller 2009).

JOINT ACTION

Another important concept in non-representational theory is that when we move (and we are always in movement), we never move as a single entity. Thrift (2008a) describes this as *material schematism* in that 'things', including us, are continually brought into relation through processes of encounter. As such, non-representational theory is concerned with *technologies of being*: "hybrid assemblages of knowledges, instruments, persons, systems of judgement, buildings and spaces" (Rose 1996, p. 132). As Anderson and Harrison (2010) suggest "the term 'world' does not refer to an extant thing but rather the context or background against which particular things show up and take on significance" (p. 8). This significance is captured as things come together, in ensembles or assemblages, to form a 'manifold of actions and interactions' – temporarily closed surfaces that produce stability.

There are several important features of *joint action* in non-representational thought. First is the question of intention. The consequence of joint action is that its outcomes cannot be fully anticipated by the individual entities it involves. Assemblages are "hybrid concretions, settings, and flows" (Thrift 2008a, p. 9). Context, or *the site*, is always an "incomplete incarnation of events" assembled within fluctuating conditions (p. 12). Individuation is ontogenetic in that processes of becoming have primacy over the states of being through which they pass: "[i]nvention is less about cause than it is about self-conditioning emergence" (Massumi 2009, p. 40). Agents are effects of struggles (Thrift 2009). Rather than possessed of a clear intent, an assemblage has a technicity, or collective character, at the heart of which is its *entelechy* (the vital force that directs it; Simondon 2009). Assemblages are not, however, completely indifferent. As Thrift (2008a) proposes, assemblages possess an open and contingent disposition.

The second feature of joint action is its dialogic nature – activity is negotiated in the moment or 'on the spot' (Thrift 2009). Encounter takes place at the surface of things, and it is through encounters that space is transmuted into context. This postulate of joint action resonates with post-structural accounts of the social, including Bruno Latour's actor–network theory and Sarah Whatmore's hybrid geographies. For actor–network theory, the social is not something already assembled but always in the process of being reassembled as actors and actants enter into, and dissolve out of, networks of relation (Latour 2007). An actor is not the source of an action but is the "the moving target of a vast array of entities swarming towards it: '[a]ction is borrowed, distributed, suggested, influenced, dominated, betrayed, translated'" (Latour 2007, p. 46). For Whatmore, hybridity involves the decentring of social agency – a "precarious achievement spun between social actors rather than a manifestation of unitary intent" (Whatmore 2002, p. 4). In this sense, the material and the social are intertwined and in constant circulation (see also the introduction to McCormack 2003).

The type of materiality advanced by non-representational theory corresponds with new materialist ontologies in the creative arts (see Bolt 2007).

32   NON-REPRESENTATIONAL GEOGRAPHIES OF THERAPEUTIC ART MAKING

Rather than harking back to notions of materialism as 'groundedness' or 'physicality', materiality here refers to the capacities of things to act and be acted upon. Matter is assumed to be common between forms of life and non-life – animate and inanimate, organic and inorganic (Anderson and Wylie 2009). Furthermore, materiality is born from turbulence – a "continual process of gathering and distribution" (p. 321). Corporeality emerges from material encounters, producing "imperatives to action which guide, imply, and ordain corporeal sensibilities" (emphasis in original; Anderson and Wylie 2009, p. 325). Put another way, *materiality inspires.*

THE PRECOGNITIVE

As already pointed out, non-representational theory trades in modes of perception that are not individualised or subject-based. Flowing from these ideas is the concept of *precognition* which Thrift (2008a), in reference to the body, describes as "a rolling mass of nerve volleys [that] prepare the body for action in such a way that intentions or decisions are made before the conscious self is even aware of them" (p. 7). In this formulation, cognition is seen as "an emergent outcome of strategic joint action for which it acts as a guidance function, monitoring and interpreting the situation as found" (also p. 7). As such, cognition is secondary to life in movement, enabling us to make only partial sense of what has already taken place.

Interestingly, the concept of life 'taking place' outside our conscious control also pervades much of contemporary cognitive science. As Maturana (2011) demonstrates:

> We human beings can make theories about the nature of life when we think that life is some property of living beings, but life is not a property of living beings, the word life only evokes or names an invented abstract entity that we claim that must be there to sustain the living of a concrete singular living being. Living does not need any theory to occur; it is the occurring of a molecular autopoietic system. (Maturana 2011, p. 146)

Maturana's argument, in a critique of representational theories of mind, is that human cognitive processes arise from the operation of human beings as living systems. We are first and foremost 'in action'; cognition is merely reflexive. Neuroscience also recognises that it is the body that gives rise to feelings and emotions, outside of our consciousness (Damasio 2000) – consciousness itself being a kind of 'user illusion', which is an imperfect reflection of the totality of our experience (Nørrentranders 1998). Furthermore, if it were not for non-conceptual processes, our concepts could not be grounded in experience and, therefore, would not possess the same meanings that they do (see Pylyshyn 2007).

This privileging of the precognitive by non-representational theory presents a unique challenge to the 'doing' of geography. If representations are always in excess of themselves, then they are "always already marked by difference and differentiation" (Doel 2010, p. 117). There is no position that can be put forward which cannot be undone. Thus, the act of representation is by nature a transformation that calls all knowledge into question. As Dewsbury (2003) suggests, we are but "false witnesses to what is there" (p. 1911). While cognition allows for the easy communication of ideas that are 'sustainable, defensible and consensual', these ideas are at odds with our delicate realities. Dewsbury (2003) provides an 'answer' to this conundrum by noting that (as researchers, academics, and philosophers) we only ever produce partial understandings of the world's 'eventhood'. We cannot hope to produce absolute knowledge, but we can commit to the production of concepts, approaches and methods that have potential to make 'coherent grasps' at the world. For Dewsbury (2003) such approaches treat thought as matter – or 'the mind in motion'. In practice, they are strivings to re-presence what we have witnessed as we communicate it (Dewsbury 2003/2010). This involves placing thought between the spaces of sensing and making sense, creating perspectives that vibrate, and giving "the right place to description" (p. 1914).

The Body

As Dewsbury (2009a) argues, non-representational theory is an ontology of sense, and sense only comes about as a "bodily event" (p. 147). As such, the capacity to apprehend eventful geographies is only made possible by a sensing body. There is a rich and diverse scholarship of the body in the social sciences from the somatic turn in the 1960s (see Turner 1996) to Foucault's (1973) *The Birth of the Clinic*, the notion of the abject body (Cregan 2006), radical feminism (Butler 1993), gender and queer studies (Sedgwick 2003), and the post-human condition (Braidotti 2013). It is not possible to do justice to the extent of this scholarship here so I will instead focus on the 'lived body' and the 'body as enactment' as they are constituted by our sense of the world (Blackman 2008).

The non-representational approach to the body is primarily concerned with the processes of becoming and the variety of ways in which "bodies are actualised and individuated through sets of diverse practical relations" (Anderson and Harrison 2010, p. 8). It is here that the concept of the lived body is brought to bear. After Merleau-Ponty, the body inhabits space and time and knows itself "by virtue of its action relation to this world" (Simonsen 2010, p. 223). The lived body incorporates the sense of the world, moving and engaging with it through a form of *corporeal consciousness* (Blackman 2008). This is different from sense perception, in its naturalistic sense, as lived experience is "located at the 'mid point' between mind and body, or between subject and object – an intersubjective space of perception" (Simonsen 2010, p. 223). Thrift puts it well when he suggests that human experience is never stable, because the "human sensorium is constantly being reinvented as the body constantly adds parts into itself, therefore, how and what is experienced as experience is itself variable" (2008a, p. 2).

The 'body as enactment' is a particularly spatial formulation of the body. Bodies are continually in the act of composing and being composed. Bodies do not remain static but are dynamic and responsive. As Manning (2007) argues (after Deleuze) to think the body in movement is to shift the question of what the body *is* to what the body can *do*. Our sense of embodiment is dependent on how our body is put to use (McPherson 2010). Bodies emerge 'in the act' of reaching *towards*, a tendency that Manning (2007) refers to as 'worlding'. Bodies are always actualising but are themselves virtual. Bodies affect other bodies and are, therefore, always in relation. Furthermore, the 'processual' body is not one that is composed of individual parts. The body in process is enacted or performed in assemblage – coupled or conjoined with other entities.

Post-structuralist theorists have made a notable contribution to the way the body is conceptualised in non-representational theory. One such postulate is that of *corporeality* (Gilleard and Higgs 2013), which refers to the body's materiality, relatively unmediated. In contrast, *soma* (or 'the somatic') refers to the body as it is 'felt', including its tactics, its positionality, the ways it reacts and responds, and how it moves (McCormack 2005). *Embodiment* refers to the body in relation – as a vehicle or medium of social agency – a merging of thinking, sensing, and relating (Tambornino 2002). Thus, while we are always corporeal in that we are 'housed' by a physical body, we experience our corporeality in a variety of ways: somatic experiences are particularly visceral, embodiment is relational. Informed by these concepts, non-representational geographers have selectively attended to the materiality of bodies (Wylie 2005), the position of bodies in Euclidean space (e.g., underground or overhead, see Garrett 2013), somatic practices (McCormack 2014), and embodied experiences (Bissell 2009), depending on the questions being posed.

In the thinking through a 'body in movement', we might also consider the body's immateriality (Blackman 2012). As Barad (2007) points out, even in a *molar* sense, the body is not bounded. We learn to 'draw outlines' that are not there. What looks like an edge is not a sharp boundary between light and dark but a series of light and dark bands – "a diffraction pattern" (p. 156). In the *molecular* sense, the body is never considered to be a uniform singularity (Deleuze and Guattari 1987). It is always multiple – formed and reformed through the movement and flux. As Grosz (1994) explains:

> subject and object can no longer be understood as discrete entities or binary opposites. Things, material or psychical, can no longer be seen in terms of rigid boundaries, clear demarcations; nor on an opposite track, can they be seen as inherently united, singular or holistic. Subject and object are series of flows, energies, movements, strata, segments, organs, intensities – fragments capable of being linked together or severed in potentially infinite ways other than those which congeal them into identities. (p. 167)

As alluded to by Grosz (1994), Deleuze and Guattari posit perhaps the most radical of all bodies – the Body without Organs (BwO). As Williams and Bendelow (1998) explain, the BwO is a 'non-productive surface' that connects assemblages with desiring-production that would otherwise be blocked by the organs' organisation into an organism. Desire passes through the body and the organs, but not through organisms. In contrast, the BwO has no organisation at all. To make oneself a body without organs is to cast off the actual body and experiment with the virtual – to allow its waves and intensities to flow through the body (Deleuze and Guattari 1987). It is these intensities and flows that are of particular interest to non-representational geographers.

AFFECT

Of all the forces with which non-representational theory grapples, *affect* is the most celebrated (Thrift 2008a). As with notions of the body, affect has a diverse set of meanings in the social sciences and humanities (Clough

36 NON-REPRESENTATIONAL GEOGRAPHIES OF THERAPEUTIC ART MAKING

with Halley 2007; Seigworth and Gregg 2010). Just as the concept of 'bodily knowledges' is now present and accepted in academic discourses, so is the notion of 'felt knowledges' or the possibility of thinking through emotion (Bondi 2005). Definitions of affect, however, still evade researchers, although that is the very point. As Bondi and Davidson (2011) argue, emotion and affect can and should defy 'sharp-edged' definition.

For the most part, non-representational theory adopts a Deleuzo–Guattarian formulation of affect (after Spinoza) understood as the capacity of bodies to affect and be affected by other bodies, be they human, non-human, animate, or inanimate (Deleuze and Guattari 1987). Affect is relational – it consists of bodily capacities that "emerge and develop in concert" (Anderson 2014, p. 9). Affect is virtual in that it is about what the body can do, and not what it is doing or has done. Affects, in the plural, are becomings. Affect, in the singular, is "essentially a pre-personal category, installed 'before' the circumscription of identities, and manifested by unlocatable transferences, unlocatable with regard to their origin as well as with regard to their destination" (Guattari 1996, p. 158). Affect is not a personal feeling or power but an effectuation of a capacity or force in and through a body as it is affected – as it acts (Deleuze and Guattari 1987).

Massumi (2002) and Thrift (2008a), as influential thinkers in geography, also adopt a pre-personal definition of affect. For Massumi (2002), affect is simply *intensity* whereas emotion is qualified intensity or "intensity owned and recognized" (p. 28). For Thrift (2008a) affect is an autonomous force that cannot be contained by the body. Accordingly, intensities 'pre-figure' encounters which then set up new encounters and so on. Affect participates in the virtual by virtue of its openness, because it "remains unactualised, inseparable from but unassimilable to any particular, functionally anchored perspective" (Massumi 1997, p. 228). Emotion, in contrast, is the intense capture and closure of affect whereas affect is always in excess of the moment of its capture and cannot be grasped alongside the perception of its capture (Massumi 2002).

It is the desire to retain an a-subjective, a-signifying conceptualisation of affect that has led non-representational geographers to draw distinctions between affect, feeling, and emotion. Anderson (2006) lays out one such theory of affect in the context of hope (one that he later revises in his 2014 book *Encountering Affect*). While acknowledging that affect is a contested term in the social sciences, Anderson (2006) agrees with Massumi (2002) in asserting that formulations of affect should not make recourse to psychology or cognition but must preserve affect's *transpersonal* nature. Although, affect has a processual logic, it is not and cannot be possessed by bodies – especially as the "human body does not involve an adequate knowledge of the parts composing the human body" (Spinoza 2011, p. 70). Affect is, however, expressed *by* bodies and is thereby fragmented into multiple registers of experience. Movements of affect, as Anderson (2006) argues, are "expressed through those proprioceptive and visceral shifts in the background habits, and postures, of a body that are commonly described as *feelings*" (emphasis added, 2006, p. 736). Feelings are an *assessment* of affect in a moment of experience as it moves through bodies. In contrast, emotion is an intimate and directly personal experience that fixes itself in words. Emotion is social insomuch as it can be articulated and folded back into more extensive networks of relations. As McCormack (2008a) explains, "[a]ffect is a kind of vague yet intense atmosphere; feeling is that atmosphere felt in a body; and emotion is that felt intensity articulated as an emotion" (p. 1827).

Although the differentiation of affect from feeling and emotion is contra to several other perspectives within the social sciences (e.g., Probyn 2010; Tomkins 1962), its implications are far reaching. Affect is always in excess of bodies – moving and circulating in and between them, emerging through and out of encounters. Thus, affect is socio-spatial phenomenon and fundamentally geographic. Although the geography of affect has attracted criticism from within the discipline (see Thien 2005) it has, at the same time, provoked diverse lines of geographical inquiry such as the therapeutics of dance (McCormack 2002), transnational experiences in and of the city (Conradson and Latham 2007), passenger mobilities (Bissell 2010), collective action and the politics of protest (Roelvink 2010), cycling (Spinney 2009), education (Kraftl 2013), surveillance (Adey et al. 2013), the atmospherics of festival spaces (Duffy et al. 2011), street performance (Simpson 2011), car mobility (Waitt et al. 2015) and human–technology relations (Ash 2013a, b). An attunement to affective life, as McCormack (2006) argues, offers "possibilities – albeit modest – for drawing out its expressive, [affective] and sometimes connective energies . . . the production of geographies that move between the many and more-than-human logics of affect, mood, emotion and feeling" (p. 332).

The concept of affective atmospheres follows on from these injunctions. As with the term 'affect', 'atmosphere' has a variety of meanings. In non-representational theory, atmospheres are a 'class of experience' that occurs "before and alongside the formation of subjectivity across human and non-human materialities and in-between subject/object distinctions" (Anderson 2009, p. 78). Atmospheres have a spatial form (spherical) – they surround and envelop bodies, human and non-human. They are not, however, reducible to an individual sense experience and cannot be possessed by bodies. Furthermore, they are sensed in a particular way – as 'supra-sensational', synaesthetic, and not sense-mode specific (Seigworth 2003, p. 81). They are ineffable, ephemeral, indeterminate, and ambiguous at the same time that they are felt and articulated in qualified emotions. Affect creates atmospheres as it moves and circulates back and forth, 'infecting' bodies like a contagion (Thrift 2008a). Atmospheres accumulate and quickly disperse in the presence and absence of bodies – they are social in origin but psychological and physical in their effects, connecting the social with the somatic (Brennan 2004; Protevi 2009).

As Anderson (2014) suggests, affects are 'always-already' imbricated in all aspects of life. Affect is "before, outside, alongside, between, across and beyond" (Seigworth 2003, p. 80). In many ways, affect is rather unremarkable. Affect is 'everything' and it is 'everywhere' – it simply exists, or is what it means to exist. Life is animated by the ordinary and made up of constant encounters between all kinds of different bodies (Stewart 2007). There is no denying the existence of affect and its force. It is integral to the moment-to-moment experience of inhabiting the temporary worlds that we, in concert with other entities, are constantly generating.

Conceptualising Space

As suggested at the beginning of this chapter, non-representational theory is spatially inflected to such an extent that it can be distinguished from other performative ontologies, epistemologies, and methodologies on this basis. McCormack (2008a) offers a clear illustration when he states:

> spaces *are* – at least in part – as moving bodies *do*. Think, for instance, of the difference between a football pitch with and without a game taking place on it. The presence of moving bodies is not only a physical transformation of the pitch: it also alters the imaginative, affective, sonic and social qualities of this space. (emphasis in the original; p. 1823)

McCormack's description draws attention to the intensive qualities of spaces in contrast to the extensive qualities of places. The football pitch is located at a place that it does not share with any other place. It is bounded. Space, on the other hand, cannot be located. It is *intensive* – you cannot contain it or 'hold it in your hand' (see DeLanda 2005). Space is lived and experienced as an embodied subject and, hence, further complicated by perspective – it is correlated with the ability to find oneself within it in order to perceive it (see Grosz 1995, p. 90). It, therefore, requires a *sensing* subject to complete it (see Dewsbury and Thrift 2005; Morris 2004).

Despite the need for space to be imagined, space is rarely explicitly theorised in the social sciences and humanities. In mathematics and the sciences, the most common understandings of space are Euclidean and Newtonian (Couclelis 1999). Massey (2005), however, asserts three alternative propositions for space. First, she urges us to think about space as a product of interrelations across a range of scales from 'the tiny' to the global. Second, she suggests that space has a contemporaneous plurality; it is a sphere of "possible existence" and "co-exisiting heterogeneity" (p. 9). Third, she argues that spaces are always open, never closed, always under construction (contra to Euclidean space). Furthermore, space is a product of relations, which are "necessarily embedded material practices which have to be carried out... always in the process of being made" (p. 9).

In the same vein, non-representational theory thinks of space in *topological* rather than *topographical* terms, foregrounding the conditions of space's emergence (Murdoch 2006). Space is a "socially produced set of manifolds" actuated by "the ensemble of movements deployed in it" (Thrift 2000, p. 19 and; de Certeau 1984, p. 117, respectively). Space is highly contingent and unsettled, being formed and re-formed in a "wide unlimited range of temporal and affective conditions, or situations" (Crouch 2010, p. 14). Space is full of creative potential. It is constituted out of materiality, objects, and movements that displace human subjectivity. Space is always becoming. It begets itself. As such, geographers have embraced the concept of 'spacing' to emphasise the mingling, diverging, non-linear means by which space is produced (Crouch 2003; Merriman et al. 2012).

In writing about space, spaces, and spacings, non-representational geographers have drawn from Henri Lefebvre's *The Production of Space*, Edward Soja's *Thirdspace*, and Gaston Bachelard's *The Poetics of Space*. Although their theoretical formulations differ, these writers take an approach to space

40 NON-REPRESENTATIONAL GEOGRAPHIES OF THERAPEUTIC ART MAKING

as social, imagined, and lived. For Lefebvre (1991) social space does not exist in of itself – it is produced by three dialectically interconnected processes, which are "doubly determined and correspondingly doubly designated" (Schmid 2008, p. 29). On the one hand he presents a linguistic or semiotic formulation of space as a triad incorporating spatial practice, representations of space, and representational space. This three-dimensional (dialectical) figure of social reality mirrors the material social production of Marx, Hegelian language and thought, and the poetics of Nietzsche (see Schmid 2008). On the other side of this double determination is Lefebvre's phenomenological formulation of space as perceived, conceived, and lived (Lefebvre 1991). Correspondingly, spatial practices are perceived materialities, spaces of representation are conceived and discursively produced, and representational spaces are lived. Finally, spaces formed by practico-social activity have multiple meanings – a material sense, a meaning in *words* and a meaning for "someone who lives and acts in the space under consideration" (Lefebvre 1991, p. 132).

Soja (1996) takes Lefebvre's theory further in proposing a 'thirdspace'. In the first instance, he articulates a *trialectics of being*, insofar as we are simultaneously historical, social, and spatial beings that create histories, geographies, and societies through collective action. Second, he posits a *trialectics of spatiality* as simultaneously lived, conceived, and perceived – a concept appropriated from Lefebvre. Thirdspace, however, is a "limitless composition of lifeworlds that are radically open and openly radicalizable ... disorderly, unruly, constantly evolving, unfixed, never presentable in permanent constructions" (p. 70). This thirdspace is differentiated from 'firstspace' (physical or empirical configurations of space which are measurable and mappable) and 'secondspace' (discursively devised representations of space). As with Lefebvre's representational space, Soja's thirdspace is lived space, although Lefebvre does not draw such sharp distinctions.

Just as there is obvious correspondence between Soja's thirdspace and the ways in which space is conceptualised in non-representational theory, Bachelard's examination of simple images of home *animates* space, bringing 'dead geographies' to life (see Thrift and Dewsbury 2000). Bachelard's (1994) work provides beautiful examples of the fluidity of space – its structures of feeling, echoes, hauntings, and shadings. As Bachelard puts it:

> the images I want to examine are quite simple images of *felicitous* space. In this orientation these investigations would deserve to be called topophilia.

They seek to determine the human value of the sorts of space that may be grasped, that may be defended against adverse forces, the space we love. For diverse reasons . . . this is eulogized space. (emphasis in the original; p. xxxv)

Bachelard's rendering of space is intimate – centring on the images of home and circling outwards, intensifying the reality of perceived objects that reverberate through space and time – a process that necessitates the substituting of 'writer' with 'creator' (Destruel 1998). Bachelard's space is imagined, his writing a poetic dreaming. It is also, however, a *topoanalysis* – the study of place as the localisation of memory. Bachelard's renderings of space find a way to stay faithful to encountering "in the immediacy of the life-worlds where it is made and re-made" (Laurier and Philo 2006, p. 353). This is at the very heart of the non-representational project.

CHAPTER 4

Performing Research

Abstract This chapter provides a comprehensive overview of the performative research paradigm as it emerged from the academic discipline of the creative arts and considers its implications for research in contemporary cultural geography. It goes on to describe the methodological approach to a research project involving practitioners of 'slow art', dance movement therapy, subterranean graffiti, poetic permaculture, and fibre art and concludes by contrasting non-representational research with ethnography.

Keywords Performative research paradigm · Geographical fieldwork · Creative methods · Emergent attunement · Research-creation

There is a sense in the reading and writing of theory that it is interminable. Theoretical writing has a rhythm and a flow that carries the passionate reader away on a stream of ideas. The evocative and seductive nature of non-representational theory is no exception. It is, in fact, a *prima facie* example – the irony being that the ideas are first and foremost about practice. In this chapter, I take up the challenge of translating non-representational theory, and the philosophies that underpin it, into a methodological approach fit for the task of providing tentative answers to even more tentative research questions. As Thrift (2000) notes, a non-representationalist approach necessitates a turn to creative praxis. Such a turn tends to reveal the often-conflictual nature of epistemology.

© The Author(s) 2017
C.P. Boyd, *Non-Representational Geographies of Therapeutic Art Making*, DOI 10.1007/978-3-319-46286-8_4

In developing a range of bespoke methods for tackling my research, I breached several research protocols. I did so deliberately, in a quest to engage with the "non-epistemic ontology-activity" that underlies all non-representational thinking (Thrift 2000, p. 216). My first breach was epistemic and relates to the appropriation of the performative research paradigm from the creative arts. Rather than appropriating these methods wholesale, I took cues from *practice-based* and *practice-led* research – two overlapping yet distinct approaches which are becoming increasingly recognised by the academy. The works of Australian art academics Estelle Barrett, Barbara Bolt, Roger Dean, Brad Haseman, and Hazel Smith are current in this regard in that they intelligently valorise processual creativity, liquid ways of knowing, and forms of data that are neither qualitative nor quantitative but performative in nature and origin (Haseman 2006; Bolt 2010; Smith and Dean 2009).

My second breach is methodological and relates to fieldwork, which on the surface may appear ethnographic. In addition to my own visual arts practice, I engaged with several other therapeutic art practices for the purposes of research, including dance movement therapy, visual art, fibre art, drain art, creative assembly, and poetic permaculture. As an adjunct to this fieldwork, I collected numerous 'sense recordings' – video, photographs, audio – which may have served as data had a qualitative approach been employed. Instead, some of these recordings formed the basis of a body of creative work, which was formally exhibited. The majority, however, served only as 'tools for thought', held in memory until they might be re-imagined at the time of writing. This approach to fieldwork differs even further from ethnography in terms of operative notions of 'self as researcher', the failure to expressly position myself in relation to 'participants', and an eschewal of reflexive note taking (see Lynch 2000). Each of these subordinate 'crimes' is justified over the course of this chapter.

The third, and perhaps most radical breach, relates to data analysis or lack thereof. It is here that Erin Manning and Brian Massumi's (2014) *Thought in the Act*, Derek McCormack's (2008b) *Thinking-Spaces for Research-Creation*, and J-D Dewsbury's (2009a) seven injunctions inspired me. Each of these researchers is somewhat Deleuzian, regarding thought as an accretion which creates effects. After Deleuze, writing can be considered as a performance that is only one small part of a wider extra-textual practice (see Thrift 2000). In this vein, my 'findings' have four alternate forms, each asserting the primacy of practice – an audio/visual form, an exhibited form, a poetic form, and a ghostly form. The audio/

visual form includes a short film (Boyd 2013) and several soundscapes, the exhibited form is discussed in the next chapter (Chap. 5), and the poetic form submitted for publication elsewhere (Boyd forthcoming). The ghostly form resides in the past, never to be presented, or is hidden away in various places on the Internet.

THE PERFORMATIVE RESEARCH PARADIGM

Frequently (albeit inaccurately) characterised as a divide, qualitative and quantitative approaches to academic research have an established history (Flick 2009). At the level of paradigm, quantitative research is more often associated with positivism whereas qualitative research is aligned with constructivism. When it comes to data collection, qualitative research employs purposive sampling and quantitative research, probability sampling – the former seeks to give voice and meaning to human (or non-human) activities whereas the latter seeks to generalise findings to a wider population. Qualitative data are predominantly textual; quantitative data are numerical. At the level of analysis, qualitative research engages with the logical process of induction, constructing knowledge grounded in data. Conversely, quantitative research engages in hypothetico-deductive reasoning, testing and refining theory in order to infer rules, laws, or models of action. While quantitative research is often considered to be 'scientific' and qualitative research as 'unscientific', this view is erroneous. Some of our greatest scientific 'achievements' were inductive, grounded in observation (e.g., Darwin 1859) whereas quantitative research methods are routinely deployed across the academic spectrum (DeFanti et al. 2015).

Over the past decade, a third research paradigm has emerged, explicitly put forward by Brad Haseman and taken up enthusiastically by many practice-led researchers in the creative arts. Known as the performative research paradigm (Haseman 2006, 2010), this approach is sufficiently distinct from constructivism as not to be subsumed by qualitative research's recent 'performative turn' (see Lincoln and Denzin 2003). The distinctive feature of performative research is that practice is not an 'optional extra' but a necessary pre-condition: "practitioner researchers do not merely 'think' their way through or out of a problem but rather they 'practice' to a resolution" (Haseman 2010, p. 147). Although naturally aligned to the creative arts, it has been noted by some scholars that performative research has the potential to make contributions across the academy (see Grech 2006).

The first way in which performative research differs from qualitative or quantitative research is in relation to the literature. Practice-led researchers 'dive in' with an enthusiasm for practice, which may or may not be guided by specific research questions. The 'problem' emerges from practice without any clear starting point. As such, performative research is intrinsically experiential: the researcher commences practising and then sees what emerges from the process. Second, practice-led researchers insist that research outputs take practice forms. Data are created, not collected (Smith and Dean 2009). Data take on symbolic, presentational forms including still or moving images, music and sound, live performance, digital code, or creative writing. As Haseman (2006) explains:

> the practice-led novelist asserts the primacy of the novel; for the 3-D inter-action designer, it is the computer code and the experience of playing the game; for the composer, it is the music; and for the choreographer it is the dance. This insistence on reporting research through the outcomes and material forms of practice challenges traditional ways of representing knowledge claims. It also means that people who wish to evaluate the research outcomes also need to experience them in direct (co-presence) or indirect (asynchronous, recorded) form. (p. 101)

There are two broad areas of artistic research encompassed by the performative research paradigm; these are the body of creative work produced and the insights that are gleaned from the process of creating the work. Together they are then generalised and written up as research (Smith and Dean 2009). The first requires a degree of technical skill that should not be underestimated (although, at the same time, the proliferation of computers and multimedia technologies has opened up the field considerably). One of the roles of the artistic researcher, then, is the dissemination of skills-based knowledge – made possible by a level of expertise in an area of artistic practice which often takes years of experimentation to attain (e.g., Dean 1989). The latter requires a kind of 'material thinking' or 'praxical knowledge' whereby the artistic researcher is attuned to the materials and processes involved in creative production, using these as a 'springboard' for thinking and understanding (Bolt 2010).

Smith and Dean (2009) advance a model of artistic research that takes both practice-based and practice-led approaches into account. Their model is iterative, with multiple entry and exit points, the key feature being its 'web-like' structure which provides the freedom for researchers to traverse from one side of the cycle to another. The cycle moves from practice-led research and the generating of research questions, through to research-led practice and the production of artwork, to the writing of academic research and contributions to theory. At any stage of the cycle, it is possible to go back or cross over. Being iterative, the cycle is repeated over and over, each time introducing variation. Smith and Dean (2009) note that choices need to be made regarding the alternate products of variation – discarding some, retaining others, perhaps even reverting to an early stage of research or modifying the very nature of the variation. Furthermore, they emphasise that to be process-driven is "to have no particular starting point in mind and no pre-conceived end. Such an approach can be directed towards emergence, that is the generation of ideas which were unforeseen at the beginning of the project" (Smith and Dean 2009, p. 23).

Nelson (2013) regards the ideas that emerge from 'practice as research' as *liquid knowing* rather than hard facts. Ways of knowing that emerge from art practice are embedded and, therefore, difficult to translate. Accounts of performative research are only ever attempts to articulate knowledge that is, at its heart, non-representational. 'Finding the words' is not impossible, however; as Nelson (2013) remarks, it is possible to describe how to ride a bike – the difference being that, with performative research, a great deal of the knowledge gains are bound up in the creative outcomes. Haseman and Mafe (2009) argue that interpretation of creative research requires reflexivity, whereas others argue that research insights cannot be manufactured but emerge, from what is an otherwise messy process as unpredictable 'shocks of recognition' that spark the imagination (Kalmanowitz 2013; O'Sullivan 2006). Goddard (2010) argues that methods of writing about creative research, such as the exegesis (Barrett 2010), must resist explanation. He likens exegetical writing as a correspondence between two practices – a creative practice and a creative 'story telling'. After Walter Benjamin, Goddard suggests that the exegesis "seeks to reveal and conceal in the same sweeping gesture". This position bears remarkable resemblance to Thrift's (2000) invoking of Wittgenstein: "[m]y work consists of two parts: the one presented here, plus all that I have not written. And it is precisely this second part that is the important one" (1969, p. 35).

From the Studio to the Field

The research for this book started with my own practice. I am not a trained artist but have, for many years, turned to art making in times of emotional distress. I do this intuitively. It was never prescribed or suggested to me that I do so. It was never done in the context of a therapy session but in solace, usually at night, and always in a state of intoxication. Prior to embarking on this research, I never questioned the 'how' or 'why' of this practice. It worked. It worked very well and helped me endure some very difficult and traumatic experiences in my life. In what was an obvious starting point, I turned to what is the most extreme example of my own therapeutic art making – a large painting I did around two weeks after a friend committed suicide and a week after a family member, who was close to her, attempted suicide three times in her wake. To my mind, the painting assisted me in expressing grief over my friend's death – something that I had felt compelled to 'put on hold' while I rushed around, trying to prevent someone I loved even more dearly from dying in the same way.

For the sake of understanding this particular event of art making, I attempted to re-enact the experience from memory. I purchased an old, manual typewriter and used it to respond affectively to the art object in the form of a poem (which was later printed onto three large canvases, forming the second exhibit in my PhD exhibition). In what became four other exhibits, I worked retrospectively with another painting, abstracting it into four 'schizoanalytic maps'. These 'maps' became the third exhibit. I went on to produce three prospective works as studies; the first, along with the photographs I took during its making, became Exhibit 1. The making of the second was filmed, thus forming a segment in the short film to become Exhibit 6. The third work arose obliquely from the research process (an unpleasant email exchange with another academic), seeing me return to the purpose for which art making has always served for me – coping with distress. This painting also became an experiment in 'thickness', forming the basis for the exhibition's seventh exhibit.

In the research's second phase, I joined with others who also spontaneously turn to art making for therapeutic and ethical reasons. The first artist was Amanda Robins who describes her work as 'slow art'. A therapist herself, Amanda first trained in visual arts, completing a practice-led PhD before taking up a second career in social work. Her work stands in stark contrast to mine: hers is delicate and considered, whereas mine is thick and messy. Hers is reflective, mine is guttural. The sessions with Amanda were to be the only ones where I did not engage in some way with the practice of another. I simply sat with her while she worked. The next practice I explored was the poetic permaculture of Artist as Family. It is the nature of this practice that it is 'all hands on deck' so this marked the beginning of a much wider exploration of practices with which I engaged first hand – for the first time and for the sake of research. I travelled with Artist as Family from Melbourne to Sydney to assist in the maintenance of a public 'food forest' which they designed and built on commission from Australia's Museum of Contemporary Art. My experiences with Artist as Family inspired me to construct a 'food forest' at home, in partnership with my own family, and as another piece of practice-based research.

The third and fourth practices both involved dance movement therapy. In the first instance, I worked with Swagata Bapat, a manager in the youth mental health sector, who once trained professionally as a classical Indian dancer. Although dance has been studied in the context of non-representational theory before, I was particularly interested in the dancer's relationship to the ground. As such, we set up a large piece of cardboard in a nearby house so that a recording device could more easily detect the sounds of Swagata's feet moving against the surface. We had three sessions together where I also recorded her dance using a Super 8 camera and asked her if she could translate her dance into a visual form. I later responded musically to five segments of sound, corresponding to the five rhythms of the practice, which I combined into a soundscape, forming the fifth exhibit in my PhD exhibition. Pieces of Super 8 footage and photography from Swagata's dancing and painting feature in the short film. Following from this, I took up classes in 5rhythms[TM] dance therapy – the form of Swagata's personal practice – for the period of one year. Close to the end of that period, the facilitators of the class helped me to organise a session where I could record the group dance, focusing again on the dancers' contact with the ground. This footage contributed to another segment in the short film.

The penultimate practice in which I took part was drain art/urban play. These two forms of 'underground art' are intimately connected. Drain art involves the practice of graffiti with spray cans and paint markers in public storm water drains. The urban play takes the form of exploration. Perhaps the most seductive aspect of drain art practice is the extent to which underground tunnels are hidden from view (see Garrett 2013). Moreover, storm water drains are unique acoustic environments, which, combined with the sound of spray-painting, produce resonances that refrain for much longer time periods than they do above ground. Part of the play, then, is a sonic play of sorts – experimentation with the acoustic strangeness of the environment. There is also a heightened sense of danger in drain art practice – physically, in that the terrain is slippery and involves a lot of unsupported climbing, but also because graffiti is a crime. Drain art is also an olfactory experience. (It really stinks down there!) Some practices of drain artists deliberately capitalise on the lack of breathable air in storm water drains by temporarily extinguishing it in flame. I had the privilege not only to be invited but also to practise alongside others who had knowledge of these environments. Three artistic contributions to the research arose from this period of fieldwork: a soundscape combined with a sculptural work that together formed the fourth exhibit in my PhD exhibition, and two segments in the short film.

The final practice in my fieldwork was fibre art. I already had a modest yarn bombing practice, taken up during the 'noughties' knitting boom in Australia. Knitting's therapeutic affordances seem underrated by academics, especially when compared to dance. Knitting is not only rhythmic but also quiet and gentle. (Dance is hot, sweaty, and exhausting.) Knitting is portable. (Dance in many contexts is socially unacceptable.) Knitting is modest. (Dance is showy, which makes the self-conscious among us very uncomfortable.) Knitting has a materiality related to the feel of fibre on the skin. It soothes. On a trip to the UK I met Lucy Sparrow, a fibre artist who works exclusively with felt, creating haptic sculptures on a monumental scale. Lucy 'sews her soul' – this is her motto. During my visit, I made a very small contribution to one of a series of 'mini-sculptures' of London landmarks that she completed on commission for *Time Out* magazine. When I came home, I joined up to the nationwide fibre art project 1000 poppies, which saw fibre artists around the country producing thousands of knitted or felt poppies in commemoration of the centenary of Australia and New Zealand's involvement in World War I. I also took part, by invitation, in the second General Assembly of Interested Parties, spending six solid hours making 'things' out of felt, performing alongside other artists, and interacting with members of the public who joined me in the making.

My research is clearly performative, although this is not a claim that a trained practitioner would feel the need to make. My fieldwork was also practice-based. My participants were not 'purposively sampled' nor were they deliberately recruited. Each of them presented themselves through chance encounters and was personally invited to take part. Amanda sent an email enquiry about the postgraduate course in youth mental health that I coordinated. Artist as Family spoke to me about their work at a friend's party. Swagata, one of my managers at work at the time, revealed her dance practice to me at a youth mental health conference after I enthusiastically shared my thoughts on a paper by Derek P. McCormack. She then put me in touch with Meredith Davies and her partner, David Juriansz, both of whom I had met the year before in a purely work context, completely unaware that they had led the 5rhythms^{TM} movement in Australia for over a decade. A former student of mine, Martin, described a night of tunnelling with an old friend to whom he later introduced me. I met Lucy Sparrow via Bradley L. Garrett who kindly agreed to host me for a few weeks at the University of Oxford in 2013, and I met Ren Walters, the instigator of the General Assembly of Interested Parties, during a 'wine break' in a research cluster meeting at the Victorian College of the Arts where we talked about music improvisation. Rather than me inviting him to my research, he invited me to his.

Doing Non-Representational Research

As Thrift (2000) argues, "in nonrepresentational theory what counts as knowledge must take on a radically different sense. It becomes something tentative, something which no longer exhibits an epistemological bias but is a practice and is a part of practice" (p. 222). It involves attending to differences in ways that encourage a re-presencing of the world we 'know' rather than the world we 'think about' (Dewsbury 2003). It involves opening up the field of geographical inquiry to the possibilities of performance – the arts of experiment *and* the art of written communication (Thrift and Dewsbury 2000). It means challenging the 'know and tell' of much of human geography and embracing failure, because we can only ever produce partial understandings of a world that simply takes place (Dewsbury 2009a).

Non-representational, performative, and affect-based research starts with the body – a sensing body in *relation*, rather than a perceiving body. This is not to say that 'I' do not see, hear, smell, touch, or taste but that it is the space between my sensing body and the world that interests me. As Dewsbury

52 NON-REPRESENTATIONAL GEOGRAPHIES OF THERAPEUTIC ART MAKING

(2003) suggests (after Deleuze), it is the world that forces us to think, encouraging us to move beyond our subject-centred understandings:

> Thinking the empirical, or the sensible, in and through the relation of affects and percepts is to constitute a domain of thought freed from the closure of representational subjectivity enabling presentations of that otherwise-unwitnessed space of emotions, desire, and faith. This is Deleuze's *transcendental empiricism*. (emphasis in the original; p. 1915)

Dewsbury (2003) describes this method of doing research (after Agamben) as a call to witness the already witnessing world. Witnessing is, thus, a form of contacting the real by intervening in it. In so doing two movements take place – the first is away from the self and towards the 'unknown' and the other is towards the self and one's own experience of the 'unknown' (Dewsbury 2003). As Sontag (1964) similarly urged, we must return to the senses in order to produce *testimony* (make use of the senses to make sense). Here, it is not only about what I sense directly but what I sense indirectly – what is felt. I do not own these intensities, however; they are shared between the world and me. Dewsbury (2003) calls this Deleuzian space, a freeing of perception from the sensible:

> [Deleuzian space is] ... a new experience of the sensible freed from point of view, both in terms of judgment and opinion and of aspect. Freeing perception, then, from one perspective to encompass several viewpoints. This is achieved in two key ways: through attention to events, and blocs of sensation. On the other hand, the space of the events, where we seize upon a fold of both activity and of passivity, is seen as an expression of "an action referred to the agent as immanent cause" (Spinoza, quoted by Agamben 1999, p. 235). On the other hand, within the blocs of sensation in embodied action ... we have the affective dimension of things. (p. 1921)

For Dewsbury (2003), this approach involves the gathering of 'life knowledge'– a 'wilder sort of empiricism', which is less about judging or reason-giving and more about *apprehending* (p. 1927). It is about being open to the 'eventhood of the moment' – the singular and unique 'flashes of encounter' that fieldwork always entails. It also challenges the widespread practice of thoroughly documenting research activity from an expert point of view. Rather, it singularises the capacity for thought in the location where it takes place. As Serres (2008) suggests, "[l]anguage is born in the emotion of encounter, words are born when you don't expect them" (p. 333).

The affective turn in the social sciences and the humanities has seen a proliferation of texts on the cultures of sense, including sensuous geographies (Rodaway 1994), haptic geographies (Dixon and Straughan 2010; Paterson 2009; Paterson and Dodge 2012), scented cartographies (Lauriault and Lindgaard 2004), sonic experience (Thompson and Biddle 2013; Smith 2000) and various 'culture readers' specifically dedicated to a single bodily sense (Bull and Back 2003; Drobnick 2006). In many ways, these texts respond to the overwhelming dominance of the visual in sociological research, but in other ways they perpetuate the myth that bodily senses are separate from one another. They also ignore the potential of what Massumi (2002) calls 'the sixth sense' – *proprioception* – the profound sense of being in the world, which might be better characterised as 'the first sense'. Serres (2008) refers to the 'sixth sense' as a unique combination of supplementary senses – heat/cold; running as breathing + jumping; lightness, weight, and speed – all of which make up the 'metasense' which he calls joy, but which might otherwise be understood as simply being alive.

For Dewsbury (2009a), sensing is the most important aspect of performative research. This type of sensing is more about 'spacing' than seeing, hearing, smelling, tasting, or touching. It is about getting "embroiled with the site and allow[ing] ourselves to be infected by the effort, investment and craze of the particular practice or experience being investigated" (p. 326). It also involves being sensitive to the ways in which our bodies are part of a wider ecology of things (Bennett 2010). The aim of performative, non-representational and affect-based research is to enliven research encounters in their re-presencing as 'findings'. And it places an extraordinary burden on the quality of this testimony to remain faithful to them (Laurier and Philo 2006).

One way to heighten the value of geographical testimony is to question some of the long-standing assumptions on which it is grounded. McCormack (2008b) suggests that two of these unspoken assumptions are, first, that space is a container in which the researcher 'thinks' and, second, that thinking is a cognitive activity involving the manipulation and recombination of the 'things' inside the container and how they are represented. McCormack argues that this leaves very little room for *research-creation*. In the act of thinking, the thinker has already become distanced from the world by uncoupling thinking from experience. Alternatively, thinking-spaces of research-creation can be likened to a

54 NON-REPRESENTATIONAL GEOGRAPHIES OF THERAPEUTIC ART MAKING

'co-intensive sensing' – the world actively participates in its own becoming before "individual agency or intentionality gets to work" (p. 3).

McCormack (2008b) goes on to argue that a range of techniques in which thinking, feeling, and doing are entwined already feature prominently in human geographical research – for example, walking, running, cycling, and dancing (or in my case, climbing, spraying, painting, digging, and stitching). The challenge is to let action inform thought and let thought inform action, to remain open and responsive to the ways that the world helps us to think, and to allow feeling, experience, and sense their rightful place in fieldwork accounts. The idea is to make more of the possibilities that experience and experiment provide for research-creation – by 'think [ing] relations in transition' and letting concepts develop their own mobility. As McCormack (2008b) explains:

> The key thing is that this is a call for participation rather than paper presentation. Blessed relief. But how might you respond to such a call? You might respond tentatively, outlining not so much a plan of action, but a sense of an ethos of openness: one guided by a notion of presumptive generosity to a world at which there are myriad sites through which to cultivate affectively imbued ethico-political dispositions. (p. 8)

ATTENDING TO FIELDWORK 'SPACINGS'

I became better attuned to spacings in my fieldwork by avoiding note taking altogether, relying instead on an 'openhearted doing' that was supplemented by visual and auditory forms of recording. Sound recording is particularly effective in this regard as a recorder can be switched on and let run. It can be 'forgotten' about, freeing up the performative researcher to take part in the 'doing' and the concurrent laying down of fieldwork memories. Photography is another thing, especially if the camera is bulky like mine. One of the ways in which I dealt with this was to be very clear about my visual focus: I was interested in practice and performance – the relation between human and non-human elements conjoined in performative acts – and I was interested in the intimacy of these relations.

This translated to three distinct types of photography. One was a limited form of 'time-lapse' in which I took rapid shots (eight frames per second) of events lasting anywhere from 10 seconds to 10 minutes. Stitched together, these photographs created a kind of 'stop frame' animation – some of which were reproduced in the short film but many of which just served as fuel for the poetic re-imaginings that came later (see Boyd forthcoming). The second style of photography was 'close up' with a pronounced depth of field. This was intended to give equal weight to the human and non-human and to highlight the texture of materials. The depth of field was to soften the 'boundary' between foreground and background. The third style, or use, of photography was in the creation of photomontages, only one of which was formally exhibited. In my research, I tried to capture movement; implied in some instances, perceptible in others as a photographic blur, and recreated in others by reanimating the images. In some of the most challenging situations, I used photography (especially rapid shutter speeds) to capture elements of my own practice. This involved doing many things in the field with one hand while holding a heavy camera in the other.

Photomontage – an arrangement of multiple photographs – is often confused with collage, an amalgam of different forms of media chosen either for their representations or material qualities (Ades 1976). Photomontage, on the other hand, disrupts space–time by visually redistributing it – randomly, if one allows the computer software to take control of the arrangement. For me, this recasts the spaces in an entirely different light – it re-singularises them. The 'sense recordings' I collected, however, should only be considered as adjuncts to a style of fieldwork that is *felt* and *sensed* before it is thought. I can think of no better way to describe the process other than a *feeling-doing*. Paramount is that which is felt, sensed, and experienced in the field but also remembered – not in detail but in weight. As Manning (2014) suggests, when we wonder the world directly, it is the wonder that remains long after our memories have faded. This was the main reason for my disavowal of note taking. As McCormack's (2002) implores:

> mov[e] beyond the apparent choice between being thoughtfully critical about a practice ... and becom[e] ethically and aesthetically responsive to the creative potentials emerging from an immersion in the pre-cognitive, pre-discursive relationalities of its kinaesthetic territories. (p. 475)

Only because it is conventional, I did give note taking 'a go' after my first session with Amanda Robins and was surprised at how derivative it was, the way in which the words stripped the fullness from the encounter despite how hard I tried to convey it in 'feeling terms'. From then on, my method did become more immersive – a 'doing' which was complemented by reminiscence rather than reflexivity (Schrag 2010) – scaffolded by thousands of photographs and over a hundred audio-recordings, the majority of which will never be seen or heard. Incisively, however, these 'sense recordings' focused on practice and not people. While I was present as a 'feeling-sensing-thinking' researcher, I was just another body (albeit a body in relation) just as the research 'participants' were also bodies.

Manning and Massumi (2014) have developed numerous strategies for research-creation arising out of workshops run at SenseLab in Montréal. Described as *thought in the act*, their approach takes "the hyphenation [in research-creation] seriously [by] seeing it as an internal connection – a mutual interpenetration of processes rather than a communication of products" (pp. 88–89). For them, research-creation is a co-mingling – an activity of relating. The work of SenseLab is focused on the potential of creative art and design practices to create new concepts. As such, it differs from traditional geographical fieldwork. There is, however, a degree of congruence between their approach and one informed by non-representational theory. Attending to the body, giving play to affective tendencies, enacting thought, embracing failure, practising immanent critique, and exploring new economies for relation are just a few examples (Manning and Massumi 2014). Notably, their work promotes an ethical and political generosity and an open invitation to collaborate.

SenseLab is 'thinking in relation' *par excellence*, but their work is more about a thinking of *human* bodies in relation. In my research, and in line with materialist and object-oriented ontologies, I wanted to lessen the distinction between researcher and 'participant' while broadening out the definition of participant to not only the people who joined me in research but to the spray can, the drain, the canvas, the soil, and so on. We were all 'participants' as we are *already-always* participating in the world. Translating the 'feeling-doing' into a body of artwork was laborious but easy. Non-textual forms of art making naturally facilitate affective knowledge translation whereas academic writing so often impedes it. Over time it became increasingly apparent to me – and through conversation with others (thank you, Thomas and Joe!) – that a written account that does justice to the 'worlding' of geographical fieldwork has to experiment with alternative ways of performing the written word. At the time of fieldwork, I did not know how I was going to do this and was not yet ready to try. At the time of writing this chapter, I am only a little clearer. In this style of

4 PERFORMING RESEARCH 57

research, the extent of faith one needs to have in the process of writing to deliver an acceptable outcome is daunting.

MEMORY AND 'SELF'

In bringing this chapter to a close, I further reflect on the importance of memory to non-representational accounts of fieldwork and consider the ways in which notions of 'self as researcher' are uprooted by non-representational theory. In keeping with this methodological approach, no definitive set of research questions is presented. Questions appear and reappear throughout the testimony to come.

Braidotti (2006) notes that in writing a two-volume study of cinema, Deleuze did not re-watch the films he wanted to discuss. He worked from memory – up to three years after he had watched a film. This method flies in the face of most academic endeavour, particularly the scientific, where fidelity to the 'source' is paramount. Braidotti's argument, however, is that working from memory promotes *transpositions* in thinking, opening up thought to the vibrant, creative, and generative interconnections that "mix and match, mingle and multiply possibilities of expansion and growth among different units or entities" (2006, p. 171). Working from memory is an unfolding of thought that is highly charged with imaginative force. What comes to the fore, she asserts, is "creative capacity that consists in being able to render the more striking lines, forces or affective charges of any given text or author … Accounting backwards for the affective impact of various items or data upon oneself is the process of remembering" (2006, p. 173). It is also a process that values lucidity (Abram 2010) and reverie (Bachelard 2005).

Bergson's (2004) notions of memory and duration are particularly relevant to this style of writing and doing research. For Bergson, memory consists of three overlapping processes – pure memory, memory-image, and perception. Perception is 'impregnated' with memory-images that materialise into 'pure memory', which is embodied. Pure memory is theoretical, because it only manifests in the "coloured and living image which reveals it" (p. 170). In contrast, the human body retains motor habits – the knowledge of acting and doing – thus possessing the potential to enact it again as a thinking being. This for Bergson, as it was for Deleuze, is human freedom. As Bergson (2004) asserts:

> the free act may be termed a synthesis of feelings and ideas, and the evolution which leads to it a reasonable evolution. The artifice of this method

58   NON-REPRESENTATIONAL GEOGRAPHIES OF THERAPEUTIC ART MAKING

simply consists, in short, in distinguishing the point of view of the customary or useful knowledge from that of true knowledge. The duration *wherein we see ourselves acting*, and in which it is useful that we should see ourselves, is a duration whose elements are dissociated and juxtaposed. The duration *wherein we act* is a duration wherein our states melt into each other. It is within this that we should try to replace ourselves by thought, in the exceptional and unique case when we speculate on the intimate nature of action. (emphasis in the original; pp. 243–244)

So what does it mean to replace oneself by thought? In one way it requires a radical shift in its conceptualisation, and in another it means surrendering to the beauty of thought in movement. The 'self' has a long philosophical history that is thoroughly explored by Charles Taylor in *Sources of the Self* – a lengthy work in which he considers the self as moral, as an expression of inwardness, as an affirmation of ordinary life, and as 'the voice of nature'. Regarding the latter, notions of self encompassed by the 'expressivist turn' see human beings as situated in a larger natural order with which they must find harmony. Taylor reckons that the "voice of nature within us" has a kind of providential significance (Taylor 1989, p. 370). This notion of self dissolves the boundaries between the ethical and the aesthetic with radical implications for 'thinking in action'. According to Taylor (1989), *making-manifest* does not mean that what is revealed is already formulated; rather it is an *a posteriori* act. This also defines what is realised as creation.

To conceive of a geographical self – or as Thrift (2008b) asserts an *allocentric* one – is to flip the ethnographic notion of self on its head. As Grene (1993) states in an extraordinary volume on the perceived self edited by Ulric Neisser, the self is inalienably ecological and that to be aware of ourselves "is to be aware not only of a product of that world but also of aspects of the world that bear on its production" (p. 112). This is more than *intersubjectivity*, which Grene (1993) argues restricts the ecological self to the realm of the human. Loveland (1993), in the same volume, argues that ecological notions of self encapsulate a theory of affordances. She, like Manning, points out that while autists fail to interpret the world from a human point of view, they still retain a strong ecological sense of self. It is the interpersonal or intersubjective self that is impaired in autism, manifesting in a struggle with pronouns (I-you) and a strange aptitude for non-subjective story telling. As Manning (2013) has argued elsewhere, the practice of 'worlding' has much in common with autism. In contrast to the helplessness of autism, however, 'worlding' is a conscious empowering of the ecological self over the intersubjective self.

My purpose in bringing the notion of self to the table is to emphasise that it is not necessary to write oneself out of geographical accounts of fieldwork in the attempt to be 'non-representational'. It instead involves a repositioning of self in relation to participants, a broadening out of what participation is, and an embracing of ecological notions of self as 'worldly becomings'. This means breaking with methodological traditions that situate the researcher at the centre of research accounts. Allowing thought to 'move' is an even greater act of surrender. For Manning and Massumi (2014), thought in movement must be granted permission to 'self-pilot'. Its potential for repetition and variation are innate. Interestingly, this is a phenomenon that several authors of fiction describe (e.g., King 2010), and one that I personally experienced in the writing of my own novel. There is an overwhelming sense in story-creation that the story writes itself. The author must 'let go' of self-as-author for this to happen. This does not mean that the author does not think but that she or he surrenders to thought – allowing it the freedom to move. It is no different from research-creation.

CHAPTER 5

Ekphrastic Geographies

Abstract This chapter focuses on the practice insights that emerged from the research project by organising them according to the techniques of painting and poetry, dancing and drawing, schizoanalytic mapping, soundscape, musical ekphrasis, photography and montage.

Keywords Ekphrasis · Schizoanalytic mapping · Musical improvisation · Durational photography · Video montage

The purpose of this chapter, and indeed this book, is to demonstrate practice knowledge. This is not easy to do, however, because so much of the "magic is in the handling" (Bolt 2010, p. 27). Done well, it involves working from the non-thought of embodied practices to a thinking through of process, taking the insights from the studio and putting them into words that provide some capture of it. This can only ever fail, but as Dewsbury (2009a) suggests, what is gained in the attempt still counts. Moreover, it counts as a particular kind of knowledge – knowledge of the affective, expressive, and non-representational kind.

The process I describe from here on is the result of a creative and emergent approach to research, one that involved a great deal of openness on my part as an arts practitioner and geographer. Commencing with studio-based explorations of my research topic, I then went out into the field to collect 'data'. On returning to the studio, I worked with these data

© The Author(s) 2017
C.P. Boyd, *Non-Representational Geographies of Therapeutic Art Making*, DOI 10.1007/978-3-319-46286-8_5

to create a body of artwork that might translate fieldwork 'findings' into forms that could be experienced *affectively*. Through trial and error, including several abandoned experiments, ekphrasis emerged as a preferred method – although, at the time, I did not have a word for it. As I later discovered, the technique has something in common with what Manning and Massumi (2014) describe as 'emergent attunement', a necessary condition for research creation.

Ekphrasis is a device for translating one art form into another by means of *apperception* (Gandelman 1991). Historically, ekphrasis was poetry that responded to a 'static' artwork such as a painting or a sculpture (Kennedy 2012). Ekphrasis can, however, take different forms such as the creation of music in response to a visual artwork or a piece of literature (Bruhn 2000) or the creation of a drawing in response to dance movement (Reason 2010). These examples are sometimes referred to as 'reverse ekphrasis'. Some scholars regard certain works of art as 'notional ekphrasis' (Bolter 2001). In these instances, an artist translates a concept or an idea into visual form. Krieger (1992) defines ekphrasis as a device to "interrupt the temporality of discourse, to freeze it during its indulgence in spatial exploration" (p. 11). Sager-Eidt (2008) argues further that contemporary modes of ekphrasis serve both cerebral and affective functions.

The process of ekphrasis is one of intense affective engagement. Therefore, employing ekphrasis as a research technique requires a theory of affect. As Seigworth and Gregg (2010) have noted, there are eight major theories of affect currently circulating in the social sciences and humanities. My research borrows from three of them. The first is the post-phenomenological notion of the body's incorporeal capacity for 'scaffolding' and 'extension'. In this conceptualisation, affect can be generated. The second is that of process-relational philosophy (after Spinoza), which links matter with a *processual* incorporeality – a feature of post-human contemporary feminism (Braidotti 2011a; Grosz 2008). In this conceptualisation, affect is always-already mediated in the world (Anderson 2014). The third is influenced by the neurosciences and quantum physics, linking the proximal senses of the body with its 'outer' context. This theory incorporates the idea that affect is transmitted in groups (between human and non-human elements of an environment) and that it can be sensed, 'felt', and perceived by the body as a force or an atmosphere (Brennan 2004).

The sections that follow are organised according to technique. Attending to technique encourages a focus on the *process* of research creation rather than its creative outcomes. In all, I focus on nine techniques, in the order that they evolved in the studio. The first is painting and poetry – the starting point being a retrospective, poetic responding to a piece of therapeutic art I made several years ago. From there, I describe the production of a prospective work in the form of a 'notional ekphrasis'. The second section describes techniques of dancing and drawing – dancing as an embodied investigation as well as drawing from the perspective of an observer of therapeutic dance. The third section describes an attempt at schizoanalytic mapping. Put forward by Guattari as an alternative to psychoanalysis, schizoanalysis is an aesthetically oriented technique of diagramming or patterning (Guattari 2013). I applied the principles of schizoanalysis to another past work of therapeutic art. Fourth and fifth are the production of two soundscapes – one produced with the intention to recreate the sonic experience of the drain art environment and the other with music making, in response to the affective flows of 5rhythms[TM] dance movement. The penultimate section focuses on montage in three forms – photomontage, stop-frame animation, and video, the latter incorporating digitised Super 8 footage. The video montage took just over six months to create and referenced each of the therapeutic art practices with which I had engaged, up to that point in time. In essence, it is a research summary.

Painting and Poetry

I no longer remember the first time I picked up a paintbrush when emotionally distressed. I figure it was some time in my early 20s. These days, anything from small works on scraps of cardboard to enormous paintings on pieces of cheap MDF are stuffed behind cupboards or left to decompose in the shed. They hold little aesthetic value, having fulfilled most of their purpose in their creation. Some of them take up space inside my house until such time as I remove them – once my 'dialogue' with them is over. Very rarely and depending on the emotional intensity of the work, I might have a ceremonial burning in the front yard.

With the aim of understanding the nature of the *spaces* created during events of therapeutic art making, my starting point was a painting I made about four years ago in a state of profound grief over the suicide of a close friend. She was 24 years old at the time. Another friend and I were expecting her to join us for dinner before a music concert, but she never arrived. While we were having dinner, she was at home hanging herself. News of her untimely death shocked many people, including a family member of mine who attempted suicide three times in the week after her death. At that time, I found myself in and out of psychiatric hospitals, offering comfort to others while trying to understand what had happened. It wasn't for another week that I made time to be alone and weep. After that, I went and bought the biggest canvas I could find and created a painting.

As an experiment in retrospective analysis, the challenge for the research was to take this painting into a 'thinking space' in a way that did not diminish its affective force. Relying on memory, I aspired to "enact the affective force of the performance event again" (Phelan 1997 in Dewsbury 2009a) but was unsure how to begin. In what Hawkins (2014) describes as the "unsaid elements of the creative process" (p. 92), I chose to type a poem about the making of this piece on a manual typewriter. I sat on the floor of my home studio with the painting and the typewriter in front of me, my goal being to convey something of the materialities and incorporeal intensities of the event, as it was re-enacted in words. The typewriter assisted in two important ways. First it enabled me to adopt and work through a sensuous disposition by employing "registers of expression that acknowledge stuttering" (Dewsbury 2010, p. 155). It also helped me 'let go' of the urge to edit what I was writing, allowing me to connect more closely with the painting rather than the poem – somewhere on the threshold between thinking and feeling (Manning and Massumi 2014). As Reeves (2013) suggests, when the prospect of editing is shelved, there is a sense that something is 'at stake' in the performance.

The idea of becoming immersed in research creation (rather than just 'thinking about' what has been created) is at the heart of the non-representational project. When I allowed myself to respond affectively to the painting, I activated memories of the event on the one hand, but on the other, I became attuned to the art object as a 'saturated phenomenon' (Marion 1998). As Mackinlay (on Marion) suggests, saturated phenomena, compared to 'common' phenomena, appear on their own terms – they cannot be aimed at, are unpredictable, and are without intentional directedness (Mackinlay 2010). Furthermore, the body is a saturated phenomenon of sorts as pain and pleasure are *auto affections*, or precognitive experiences, that cannot be aimed at either. Allowing the visible to be revealed and to experience this viscerally through typewriting became a kind of 'ritornello game' – at once transversal, gentle, and novel (Guattari 1995; McCormack 2008a; Whitehead 1978).

I did not know what my hands were doing and then some-*thing* appeared on three A4 sheets of paper. At least that's what it felt like. Nonetheless, there was a sifting through of experiences, emotions, and memories for those that might shed light on the activity. The resulting poem is a mixture of emotion, thought, movement, and materiality as they came into relation with one another in the creative act. The process of creating the poem was an enactment of 'the refrain' (McCormack 2014). I was able to take several ideas forward from this experiment – most importantly that an attunement to affect does not necessitate a distancing of emotions and that these can be named (Colls 2012; Simonsen 2010; Thien 2005).

This poem was just the beginning of my 'making sense' of the non-representational geographies of therapeutic art making. In preparation for exhibition, I had each A4 sheet printed onto a 1000 × 1500 mm canvas such that each individually typed letter was about 50 mm in height. As one visitor to the exhibition wrote in the visitor's book: "[t]he stutter resonated at first, then the typeface. The ambiguity/undecidability of paint/poison/wine. Eventually I felt an undefined affective response, disturbed by a shadow" (Anonymous 2012; used with permission). Thus, audiencing of the work was another refrain in the creative process. Spatialising the original work by creating another became an ontogenetic process whereby I was 'becoming' as a researcher at the same time that the evolving artwork was tracing a movement of affect.

Taking what I had learned from the first experiment, I prepared to embark on another aesthetic experiment – to practise 'emergent attunement' through the production of a new painting. Because I wanted to understand the therapeutic-ness of the event, I waited until such time as I felt the need to paint. Preparation involved purchasing pigment, impasto, gel medium, and a large square canvas. A particularly turbulent time at work, combined with an empty house, provided the right circumstances and impetus to begin.

I always paint with the canvas lying flat on the floor. This is because I like to get 'up close'. There is a lot more physical movement in painting horizontally – circling the canvas, reaching over and across it. I like to use a lot of paint, and so painting horizontally helps to keep paint in place while it dries. For this painting, I mixed structural acrylic paint with impasto and gel medium. Impasto is a very thick, viscous substance, whereas gel medium adds gloss to the paint. In choosing the mediums with which to work, I was also setting the parameters of the affective engagement. As McCosh (2013) argues, "matter informs the artist throughout the creative process" (p. 129).

Working with thick mediums does not lend itself so easily to brushwork. Instead, I use palette knives. Artist's palette knives come in various thickness and lengths and usually have a flexible tip. Moving, dispersing, overlapping, scraping, marking, and smoothing over paint with a palette knife will achieve different effects. Using a thick, structural paint makes it possible to move quickly and roughly with some resistance. Doing so creates peaks and troughs in the surface – a topography of sorts – which can be moulded and reshaped as the painting progresses.

After mixing paint, I pour it in large sections, or blocks of colour without form. Once there is ample medium on the canvas I 'get to work'. The process, from here on, changes. The preparation of paint is a thoughtful and deliberate act, whereas the activity of painting is not. Bolt (2010) describes it as 'working hot'. I like to think of it as a kind of 'sensory melting'. Either way, the artist's body and the materials start to merge. McCosh (2013) argues that distinctions between the mind, body, and environment are extinguished in creative acts. For me, this is an act of surrender – a complete and unreserved surrender to process and 'the event'.

O'Sullivan (2006) and Zepke (2005) argue that art making has the ability to de-territorialise the subject. In this sense, the artist uses the incarnate or material components of practice to construct an image of thought. This works by opening up a 'plane of consistency' which frees the artist to explore the creative and affirmative potential of practice – the potential to 'see' the world differently. O'Sullivan (2001) characterises this as the *aesthetic impulse*: "a desire for an affirmative actualization of the virtual and to move beyond the already familiar (the human), precisely a kind of self-overcoming" (p. 129). Creating a painting as a 'notional ekphrasis' enabled me to experience this more consciously.

As Collins (2014) suggests, "[w]ords might possibly be used to describe or narrate what happens during the creative process, but materials have voices of their own" (p. 148). There is a sense of responsibility on the part of the artist to 'listen' to what the materials are saying. The difficulty with this painting, initially, was the contrived way in which I attempted to reflect on the process while it was taking place. Engaging the reflexive mind closes down the creative process in a similar way that note taking closes down apprehension. I had the typewriter next to me, took breaks from painting to type reflections, and took numerous photographs of the painting in its initial stages, which necessitated painting with one hand. While this gave me the 'data' that I needed for my research, it was so contra to the creative process that I had to abandon it so that I could finish the painting. Thus, from this second experiment I learned more lessons to take forward into the field. The first was the importance of keeping reflexivity at bay. The second was that in giving primacy to practice one must abandon oneself to chaos. Post-event theorising has its place, not as reportage, but as part of a polyrhythmic "distribution of the sensible" (Manning and Massumi 2014, p. 113). The knowledge held in the painting is greater than anything I could put into words.

Once finished, I titled the painting *Sturm und Drang* and described it, at exhibition, as a 'notional ekphrasis' on the non-representational geographies of therapeutic art making. 'Sturm und Drang', translated from German, means 'Storm and Drive' (or 'Storm and Stress'). The term has been used to describe the cultural turn in German literature and music in the late seventeenth century that gave free expression to emotion. This seemed appropriate in terms of describing its process and aesthetics. Although the painting is non-representational in form, when I look into it, I see stormy weather. At exhibition, many visitors saw stormy seas, with one visitor noting in the visitors' book, "I was most drawn to *Sturm und Drang* – I felt drawn into the sea of textures and expressiveness, viscerally" (Anonymous 2013; used with permission). As such, its non-representational form seemed to resonate with visitors. As Deleuze (2000) suggests, the signs of art are immaterial and integrated into the work: "[t]his is why art is the finality of the world, and the apprentice's unconscious destination" (p. 50). Alternatively, as Shipp (1922) puts it,

> Abstract form is the embodiment of an artist's ideas about a thing, freed from the re-iteration of its concrete appearance, thus revealed the more intensely the dynamics which went into its creation, the laws which govern its existence, its structional and emotional interest, and by these means the significance which it has in the scheme of the universe. (p. xii)

In summary, the time spent in the studio before embarking on my geographical fieldwork marked the beginning of a commitment to process that is necessary when employing non-representational methodologies. It is an ethical commitment to "learning to become affected" (McCormack 2008b, p. 9).

DANCING AND DRAWING

The aim of my geographical fieldwork was to extend my exploration of therapeutic art making beyond my own practice. By incorporating the practices of others into the research, I was also able to appreciate the different environments in which ethico-aesthetic activities take place. In being new to a practice and engaging in it for the first time, I had the benefit of 'fresh eyes'. Each encounter was vividly novel. This helped when it came to maintaining the open and sensuous disposition that one must cultivate to engage fully in non-representational research.

Each contact with a new practice involved a period of observation, after a request to a practitioner to allow me to witness his or her practice. Rather than a passive form of observation, however, it was an opportunity to foster a relation between us by intervening in what would otherwise be the practitioner's private endeavour. As such, my observation involved parallel processes of composition – a shifting between drawing, typing, filming, recording, and listening – across durations and as the fieldwork encounters unfolded. It was about finding ways to relationally respond to an activity by attempting to capture a semblance of it. In some cases, I invited practitioners themselves to respond, ekphrastically, to their own practice as another aesthetic experiment.

To recap the method, one of my first forays into geographical fieldwork was an encounter with dance movement therapy and a private session with Swagata Bapat, who was once a professional Indian dancer and now a practitioner of 5rhythms^{TM} dance therapy. Although it is not the only way to practise, she decided to dance a 'wave' in our research sessions – a continuous dance which moves through five rhythms of music: flowing, staccato, chaos, lyrical, and stillness (Roth 1998). Unlike a facilitated class, when practised privately, the dancers choose their own music to match their understanding of the rhythms. Music that supports 'flowing' might be a slow ballad or an *andante* from a piece of classical music. Music that supports staccato might be a 'punchy' rock song. Music that supports the chaos rhythm often has a strong and rapid 'drum and bass' line, such as electronic music that has a 'tribal' quality. Lyrical involves a slowing down to a more moderate pace, with 'pop' style songs that are cheerful. Stillness makes use of very slow, droning, or melodic instrumental music.

As Manning (2009) suggests (after Dalcroze), rhythm is not "solely of the ear" (p. 131). Rhythm calls for a muscular and nervous response from the body – it permeates the body, 'becoming-body'. Witnessing the becoming-body through active observation is an exercise in consistency. Swagata's movements resonated within me as she responded relationally to the music and to the tension of my busyness. We allowed ourselves to be mutually present in the event, responding in alternative ways that created a relational synthesis. The sensing body in movement is enchanting. Her movements impelled my movements. We improvised. What we felt is what Manning (2009) describes as the incipient potential to move which opened us both up to movement as *pure plastic rhythm*. In process, I was provoked to 'wonder the world directly' (Manning 2014).

To draw the dance is to be perplexed by movement. Reason (2010) calls it 'kinaesthetic empathy', which is not expressible in discourse. It is an act of transposition that invites the spectator to access something new (Reason 2012). In drawing the dance, the incipience of action is transferred to the hand. The hand allows itself to become displaced by the affective tonalities of rhythm, sketching out a shape of affect on the page. This creates visual knowledge of how it feels to move. My ekphrastic responses to Swagata's dance took the form of charcoal drawings on a large sketch pad. These drawings responded to the vectors of Swagata's movement – her strivings to extend her body beyond its apparent physical boundary. Her limbs stretched outwards and up while her feet incessantly pounded the ground. As such, my drawings looked like a vortex, sucking force in and expelling it out and down – into the earth in an expression of 'grounding'. In grounding, the body becomes a part of the floor allowing a pure body of sensation to emerge. After Deleuze and Guattari (1987), body and ground become a functional assemblage – an autonomous composition of sensation which is itself a work of art.

Our next session together was for the purpose of 'data collection'. Swagata wore headphones so that I was unable to hear the music. We sourced a huge piece of cardboard to use as a dance surface. An audio-recorder captured the sounds of her feet connecting with the ground, while I moved around her with a Super 8 camera. She danced with eyes closed. Back in the studio, I listened back to the audio-recordings. With a selection of artist's chalks and paper, I attempted to draw the rhythms. Rather than five, I ended up with seven – one corresponding to each of the five as well as one for the fractious transition between 'flowing' and 'staccato' and the other for the 'becoming-animal' that emerges out of the 'chaos' rhythm. Roth (1998) characterises 'flowing' as feminine and 'staccato' as masculine. In what are referred to as gateways, the path to 'flowing' is in the feet, whereas the path to 'staccato' is in the hips. It is perhaps the most abrupt transition in the 'wave', but one that opens out to the abandonment of the 'chaos' rhythm. Dancing 'chaos' is exhausting. It is in this exhaustion that the body begins to express itself sexually, in gestures and movements that originate deep in the pelvis. This is the intensification of the cosmological forces of the earth that give rise to the new, akin to the power of sexual selection (Grosz 2008). The dancer embraces this excess for the sake of sensation itself.

For the third session, I came prepared with a black, primed canvas and some paint. Swagata agreed to attempt an ekphrastic painting of her own dance. We recorded the sound of her movement again, but this time I sat quietly allowing her to 'centre' herself. On completing the wave, she immediately went to the canvas and picked up a brush. We didn't exchange words. I picked up a camera set to a rapid shutter speed – eight frames per second. She started in the centre with red, roughly applying thick blobs of paint with a palette knife. From within the red centre, she then painted radiating lines of yellow, which extend past the red towards the four corners of the canvas. She broke the lines by dotting them with a brush, stretching them out still further. At the perimeter she applied blue paint, connecting the yellow lines with more blobs of colour. Taking the yellow on the end of her fingers, she swirled through the blue creating spirals of yellow that became green at the edges. She continued in this vein, drawing more yellow lines that spread out from the centre and terminated in more spirals. She completed the painting by converting some of the spirals into exploding stars.

And so at the end of our three sessions together, we had three examples of ekphrastic work translating the carnal knowledge of dance movement into visual form. The series of charcoal 'vector diagrams' pointed to the therapeutic-ness of grounding. The series of chalk drawings, in response to the sound of the dance, revealed the tension of moving from 'flowing' to 'staccato' and the intensification of sexual energy that emerges out of 'chaos'. The ekphrastic painting accentuated the phenomenon of 'extension', a contacting of the virtual, an expression of feeling – a diagram of becoming.

SCHIZOANALYTIC MAPPING

Convinced of the power and utility of ekphrastic drawing, I went back to the studio to attend to another retrospective work. Titled 'Aftermum, Aftermath', I had done the painting some years earlier following a difficult visit from my mother. Unlike the painting I had made in response to grief, this non-representational painting had consciously evaded me. Inspired by McCormack's (2005) deployment of the 'diagram', I produced four 'schizoanalytic maps' of the painting. These then became tools for thought so that I might make better sense of the therapeutic value of the work. This method also helped me to better appreciate the art object in the way that Guattari understood these sorts of paintings as being: "like a symphony articulating all the levels of your 'self', simultaneously exploring and inventing it through painting" (Guattari in Genosko 2002, p. 62).

For Guattari (1995), subjectivity is plural and polyphonic. The unconscious strives towards subjectivation – an *autopoïēsis* or a processual creativity through praxis. Although not exclusive to art making, Guattari privileged arts practice for its ability to de-territorialise the subject. It is in the smooth, liminal spaces of creativity that lines of flight occur, which enable or diminish affective capacities. Ethico-aesthetic practices operate transversally (or non-hierarchically) to produce a praxical opening to the virtual. In the process of making, the artist cultivates an *ethos* – an openness to the onflow of the world combined with a sense of self as 'prospectively unfolding'. The 'making' is not only a making of a work of art but a kind of 'self-making' as well as a 'making sense' (Collins 2014; O'Sullivan 2010).

McCormack (2005) argues that the affective power of practice is given conceptual consistency by adopting a diagrammatic style of thinking. Diagrams, in this sense, are maps that connect different lines of affective force. In applying diagrammatic thinking to dance, McCormack (2005) produced diagrams of corporeal movement – what Massumi (2002) calls *biograms*. In contrast, the 'schizoanalytic maps' I produced in the studio were abstractions taken from the creative product of an event of subjectivation. This is different from a biogram in that it does not correspond to the movement of the body but to a movement within the self. It is 'schizoanalytic' in that it is a method for effecting a 'break' from self to the plane of consistency where becoming takes place. It is 'mapping' in that it creates a cartography of the self – a meta-modelling of chaotic processes that move the self towards bifurcation. Whereas McCormack (2005) sees his diagrams as mapping the relations between "kinaesthetic movement, social and cultural transformation, and architectures of performative potential" (p. 143), I see my abstractions as spatialising affect, 'lifting' it out of a static work so that it can be apprehended. In both cases, however, our diagrams respond to the affective power of the non-representational.

In terms of artistic process, I created the four schizoanalytic maps by filtering a digital photograph of the painting in Adobe Photoshop CS5.1, a commercial software program for manipulating images. I simply applied preset filters at random until I achieved a result that 'spoke'. Each map was greyscale, filtering out the colours of the painting. This is not to suggest that colour does not play a role in the work, only that it distracted from the painting's less obvious and more rhizomatic elements. The first image highlighted the figure-ground, emphasising 'shape'; the second suggested 'movement and flow', the third filter inverted the image invoking notions of territory and entrapment; and the fourth highlighted the painting's textural qualities. The first map 'pulled out' a black figure, placing it on a plain, white background. The figure resembles a hydra – a mythical creature – but instead of multiple heads, the figure has multiple tails or tentacles. In the second map, the creature appears to be 'swimming' in stagnant water, surrounded by 'algal blooms' that hold it in place. In the third, the image looks fossilised, pressed into the earth. In the fourth, the image is softer and more gently enveloped by its surroundings.

Collins (2014) describes schizoanalysis as "'at once transcendental and a materialist analysis', seeking the transcendental conditions of experience and then defining these conditions according to a materialist immanence" (p. 65). In terms of process, the first task of schizoanalysis is to 'cleanse' the unconscious by reorienting it towards desiring-production. The second is to discover the nature of the desiring-machines of our unconscious mind, the part that desires connection to others. The third is to 'separate the psychic investments of desire from the psychic investment of interest' – the social from the familial. In this way, schizoanalysis achieved through art making *counter-actualises* the 'accident' of being, freeing the ego from its wounds by releasing its energy and putting it to ontogenetic work. Collins (2014) calls this 'transformative therapeutics' – the immanent sense and transformation that arises from the creative process. My own schizoanalytic experiment revealed something abstruse about the particular piece of art on which it was based – I had painted a trapped inner 'monster' attempting to swim free. Unbeknown to me prior to the experiment, the painting had diagrammed an event of radical subjectivation and the engendering of new existential territory.

SOUNDSCAPE

Back to the field and I was keen to explore styles of therapeutic art making that might provide contrast to the 'genteel' practices of painting and dancing. An invitation to accompany someone into an underground storm water drain to conduct graffiti presented the ideal opportunity to expand the research into another realm. Drain art as a practice is part visual art making and part urban play. As a form of visual art making it could be considered as 'minor art' in that its materials – aerosols, drip markers, and scrawlers – and its canvas, the tunnel wall, are a de-territorialisation and re-territorialisation of the 'major' (O'Sullivan 2005). The aspect of urban play in drain art practice is performed in the spirit of *urbex* – a practice that seeks not to vandalise or destroy but to discover and reveal (Garrett 2013). Thus, the core components of drain art practice are at odds with one another. The art leaves a mark deliberately intended for a very exclusive audience of fellow 'drain walkers'.

Neither the government body that maintains Melbourne's network of drain tunnels (Melbourne Water) nor the organisation which promotes drain exploration in Australia (The Cave Clan) advertise the location of drains. As the outlets are usually hidden from view, it is only possible to gain access to a drain by being invited or by accidently stumbling upon one. In terms of art practice, there is a similar gradation from tagging, to 'throw ups', to 'wildstyle' or more intricate, colourful pieces that one sees in graffiti that takes place above ground (McDonald 2001; Young 2014). The key difference, however, is that subterranean graffiti has a much more limited 'public'. Drain artists perform for themselves and each other.

Drains in Melbourne carry storm water away from the kerbside. Although they do not contain sewerage, the water is not treated and, therefore, the drain environment has a slightly unpleasant smell. One only has to venture a short distance into a drain before the available light is not sufficient for navigating the environment. As such, drain artists and explorers usually wear head torches and carry additional light sources with them. The diameter of a drain is at its maximum at the point where it connects to external waterways, but for the most part there is plenty of head clearance for artists and explorers to move about freely. Standing or walking in a drain involves either placing a foot on each side of the flowing water or walking directly in the stream. Drain artists carry materials in buckets which can be set down on the drain's curved surface so that they are not lost in the current. The most difficult part of navigating a drain is its camber and the fact that water flows through its lowest point. Rather than sloping, drains are usually 'stacked' so that one might travel for several metres before encountering a 'subterranean waterfall' at the point where two drains intersect. In order to proceed, practitioners climb up old, rusty ladders loosely connected to the drain wall by metal chains, balancing buckets and torches in both hands. In doing so, they get drenched with water so that for the rest of the draining session their clothing is smelly and wet through.

The therapeutic-ness of drain art practice partly arises from the slipperiness of its terrain (evoking a sense of adventure) as well as the restriction of the visual sense that serves to heighten the remaining senses. Rapidly flowing storm water, the hissing of the spray paint, and the clunking of cans as they are thrown back into plastic buckets combine and ricochet to produce a 'working' environment that is completely dominated by sound. It is not uncommon for drain artists to offer up their human voices to this non-human symphony as a kind of mimetic encounter.

Perhaps the most remarkable aspect of 'draining', however, is the unique melding of person and environment that goes beyond states of awareness involving sight and sound and into "the world of proprioceptive transformation brought on by extrapersonal loci" (Thrift 2008a, p. 84). In the drain, there is a strong sense of being underneath, running in parallel to, a world that is unfolding above. There is a 'given-ness' to this environment that makes the practitioner feel like an interloper. The odd locations where the two worlds intersect provide opportunities to view the world above from a different perspective; for example, on arriving at a grate that runs under a busy highway, it is possible to lie down and look up at the sky while being 'run over' by the traffic. Drain art practice is "a call to creativity, a call to become actively involved in various strategies and practices that...allow us to produce/transform, and perhaps even go beyond, our habitual selves" (O'Sullivan 2007).

The capacity for sound to interpellate the body into space is of great interest to sonic geographers, sound artists, and philosophers (e.g., Duffy 2012; Duffy et al. 2011; Gallagher 2014; Gallagher and Prior 2014). Sound is spatio-temporal in that it is 'pressure in the air' (or amplitude) over time. Measured in space–time, sonic vibration can be detected as a wave, but the wave itself is made up of complex, irregular elements such as "harmonic oscillations, pure tones, timbre-less notes of various volumes and pitches all sounding together" (Evens 2002, p. 172). Unlike vision, which supplies an illusion of continuity and stability over time, sound is a dramatic display of the world's 'eventfulness'.

Gallagher and Prior (2014) argue that "audio media lend themselves to empirical work on aspects of geography that are hidden, fleeting, beyond or at the periphery of everyday awareness...highlight[ing] overlooked and intangible aspects of environments...magnifying liminal features of places" (p. 5). Sound recordings are routinely employed in the production of audio documentary as naturalistic sounds overlaid with music and narration designed to 'educate' the listener (see Ferrington 1994). Contemporary methods of soundscape production are more akin to the arts of experiment – what Gallagher and Prior (2014) refer to as 'sound writing' or the 'sounding of space'. This involves working with sound in creative ways to produce sound works with the capacity to provoke "mimetic engulfment and activated spectatorship" (Thrift 2008a, p. 86) at a level in excess of representation.

Gallagher (2015) suggests that there are four main uses of field recordings in geographical research. The first is 'the nature style', the second 'soundscape', the third 'acousmatic', and the fourth 'sound art'. In order to produce a sound work that would translate the non-representational geographies of drain art practice in fruitful ways, I enrolled soundscape as a technique. According to Gallagher (2015), soundscape mingles human and non-human sounds producing a "lifelike mimesis of the recorded field '…[in a] thickening, melding, juxtaposing, or fusing of acoustic space-times–a form of bricolage or hybridization" (p. 566). In the production of a drain art soundscape, I did not rely solely on the sonics of the environment to achieve this. I layered audio-recordings over one another to accentuate multiple dimensions of the fieldwork encounter. For instance, the sound of spray paints, the murmur of voices, the roaring of a subterranean waterfall, the sounds of footsteps as they splash through the water, the crash as paint cans hit the bottom of a plastic bucket, the harmonics of 'drain singing' were 'folded' over one another to produce a sense of space designed to invite a curious listener in. In this regard, the soundscape is more performative than representational.

The audiencing of soundscape is particularly important as it is in the 'playback' that the work is performed: the 'data' of field recording becomes movement through vibration. Through vibration, sound is embodied by listeners in that they listen with their entire being (Nancy 2007). Furthermore, sound is invisible, which serves to incite listeners to enter into and explore a soundscape's construction (Voegelin 2014). The soundscape I produced from field recordings of drain art practice was 10 minutes in length. At exhibition, it was stored on a first-generation iPod shuttle on a lanyard, looped, and then connected to a set of noise-cancelling headphones. The listening apparatus was hung from a 3-metre sticker-bombed pole set in 20 kilograms of concrete – the sticker comprising a photograph of a piece of drain art made during one of the fieldwork sessions. Visitors to the exhibition on encountering the exhibit were able to have a somewhat private experience of the soundscape by blocking out the surrounding noise and engaged their 'auditory imaginations' (Idhe 2003). Of all the exhibits, this was the most remarked upon. Visitors not only found the soundscape intriguing but further indicated that it created a unique sense of space; as one visitor commented in the visitors' book, "the voices in the space reminded me of a call and response – a sense of play. I felt like I could hear joy and sense these bodies in the place and, I guess, with the place – back and forth, here and there – and also, I felt like there was a space for me as the listener. I wanted to be led in by the voices and the spray painting" (Anonymous 2014; used with permission).

The main insight gained from the practice of drain art, and the production of a soundscape from audio-recordings made in the field, was the affective power of sound. The vibrations that are created, as sounds bounce off surfaces and penetrate bodies, are surprisingly potent (Grosz 2008). The work also enabled me to understand how some features of therapeutic space are 'given' to us by the world. The environments in which we choose to practise can impact us in unpredictable ways.

MUSICAL EKPHRASIS

The work on the 'drain art soundscape' helped me to develop techniques for 'sound writing', which I was then keen to apply to other aspects of the research. I was cognizant that the foray into soundscape was technically not an application of ekphrasis as method, so in an attempt to continue this set of aesthetic experiments, I considered what a sonic ekphrasis might be. To explore the concept, I returned to the audio-recordings of 5rhythms^{TM} dance made the year before. Through attentive listening, I had created a series of ekphrastic drawings as a response to the sounds of the dancer contacting the ground. In returning to these field recordings, I wondered what might be gained from attempting to respond to them affectively with sound.

Although much is written about musical ekphrasis (composers responding to painting and poetry; see Bruhn 2000), I could find no guideposts for responding to practices with sound. Instead, I found inspiration in Hayden Lorimer's notion of 'make-do methods'. For Lorimer (2010), "'make-do methods' are not pre-planned but 'fallen upon', involving a degree of 'faith…in our human abilities to perceive them'" (p. 258). They are "collagist and 'chthonic'" in character and a bit surreal (p. 259). In creating my first sonic ekphrasis, I took on Lorimer's (2010) provocation to combine a receptive attitude of mind with heightened powers of observation and an openness of manner.

In adopting a 'make-do method' to sonic ekphrasis, I also employed the principle of 'readiness to hand' (Bolt 2011). After Heidegger (1962), Bolt (2011) suggests that the use of 'tools' in art making is different from the 'every day' use of tools out of habit. It creates a "clearing, a space ... [o]ur handling or dealings with entities in practice offers a special form of (in) sight ... a *poietic* rather than an enframing revealing" (emphasis in the original, p. 89). We come to know tools as 'ready-to-hand' but, in their use, they affect a withdrawal towards a world in which the work they do comes to the fore. Bolt (2011) suggests that in the process of art making, tools become grafted to the artist. Artists work in relation with the tool, rather than gaining mastery over it. In order to produce an ekphrasis through musical responding, I seized every music-making 'tool' in my house: this included my concert flute, cello, guitar, tin whistles, bongo drum, piano, tambourine, rhythm sticks, and musical chimes. I lacked the confidence in the beginning to use the entire suite of instruments, opting instead to focus on technique. (I made use of the full range of instruments later, in producing a series of ekphrastic pieces to accompany the short film – the final piece in this body of creative work).

I cannot play the guitar much past a few basic chords. Therefore, improvising with an instrument meant being attentive to its sounds and vibrations. Rather than thinking about the sounds of the instrument, however, my thoughts turned to the sounds and memories of Swagata's dance. In preparation, I selected five segments of audio, each of approximately a minute in length, corresponding to each of the five rhythms. I 'stitched' these together electronically using Final Cut Pro 10 software, cross-fading the audio between each segment. After converting the file to a portable file format, i.e., mp3, I loaded it onto a separate player freeing up the laptop to record the musical ekphrasis. I then listened to the field recordings with headphones while letting my hands and ears respond to what I was hearing. This not only involved plucking and strumming strings, but also vibrating them with a cello bow, or knocking against the instrument's body.

In contrast to representational thinking, improvisation begins with attunement – a praxical opening. As Crawford (2013) argues, "attunement is a way of thinking about some thing that seeks to be open and connected to said thing" (p. 4). This style of thinking is 'gut-level' and momentary rather than analytical or rational. Heidegger described three ontological characteristics of attunement. The first is its 'throwness' – being thrown into a situation or into the world. The second is its 'directedness' towards something (disclosing the world), and the third is elucidation – a movement towards the self where one is affected or moved (Heidegger 1962). Durant (1989) suggests that musical improvisation is simultaneously liberation, discovery, and dialogue. It is liberating in that it is an 'unravelling' of form (Crawford 2013); it is discovery in that it is a reconstituting of the 'old'; and it is dialogue in that it is an exploration of relationships between musicians or between musicians and audiences.

My intention with the sonic ekphrasis was two-fold – the generation of praxical knowledge and the communication of that knowledge to willing listeners. As Crawford (2013) suggests, musical improvisation seeks to transform. Listening is transformative, because it is a search for meaning. According to Nancy (2007), to *hear* is to understand the 'sense' but to *listen* is to 'stretch the ear' – to always be on the edge of meaning, a meaning that is only found in resonance: "meaning and sound share the space of a referral, in which at the same time they refer to each other, and that, in a very general way, this space can be defined as the space of a *self*" (p. 9). Thus, to communicate through sound is to resonate from *self* to *self*, from *I* to *other* – "the sound of sense is how it refers to *itself* or how it *sends back to itself* or *addresses itself*, and thus how it makes sense" (emphasis in the original; Nancy 2007, p. 9).

In terms of praxical knowledge, the production of musical ekphrasis involves a complete abandonment of the linguistic and total embrace of the power of the non-representational. It is an abstraction of thinking-feeling, without words, which stimulates the imagination of the listener (Priest 2013) – not so much as a transmission but as a *sharing* of feeling, an intensely expressive capture of the flux of experience that constitutes the world. Imagination always terminates in a concept (Massumi 2011). Music, in particular, breathes life into thinking by infusing imagination with sensation.

Photography and Montage

In sympathy with the rest of the project, photography provided another opportunity to experiment with an expressive medium. The following pages make room for a small selection of the thousands of photographs taken.

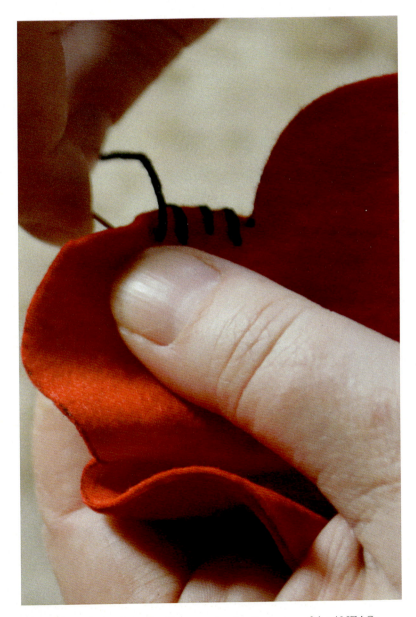

Stitching – The fashioning of a felt poppy for the Centenary of the ANZACs

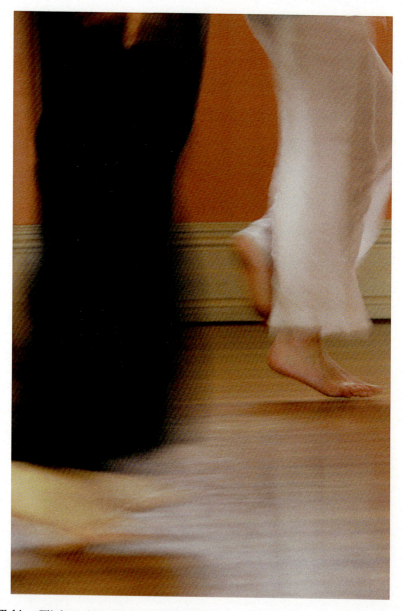

Taking Flight – A moment in a 5rhythms™ dance class when two dancers leave the ground at the same time

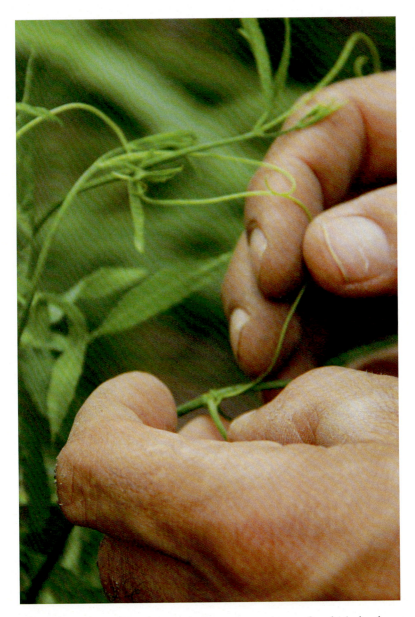

Entraining – An act of poetic permaculture where a human hand winds a banana passion fruit plant around an upright support

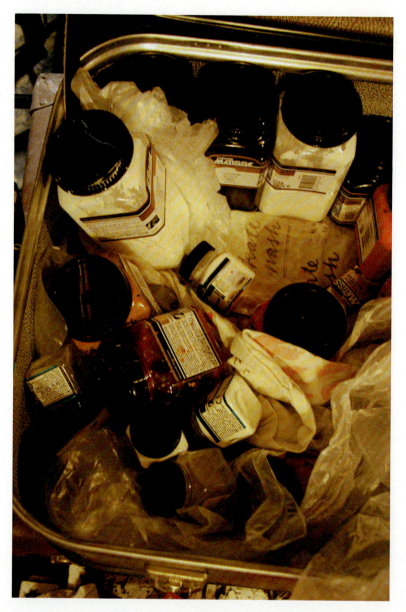

Paints – An example of object-oriented photography in which inanimate materials become portraiture

5 EKPHRASTIC GEOGRAPHIES 83

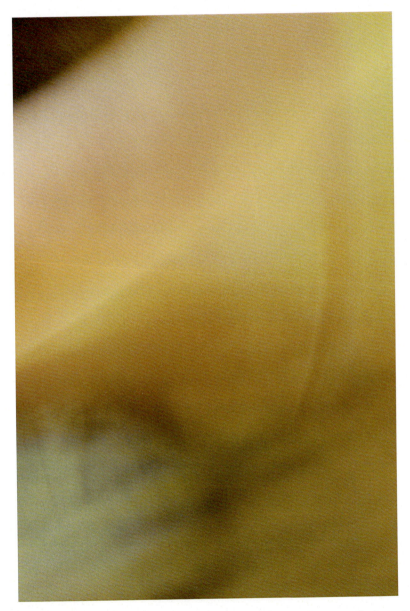

Trace – An example of durational photography where the movement of a dancer's arm and hair blur to create an image without subject or object

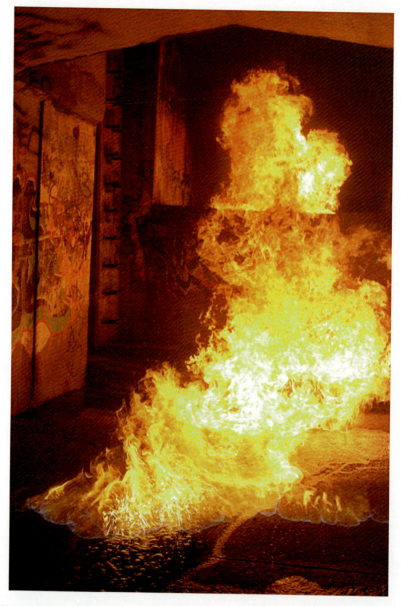

River of Fire – One of several photographs, taken during an event of 'fire-setting' in a storm water drain that went into producing a stop-frame animation

5 EKPHRASTIC GEOGRAPHIES 85

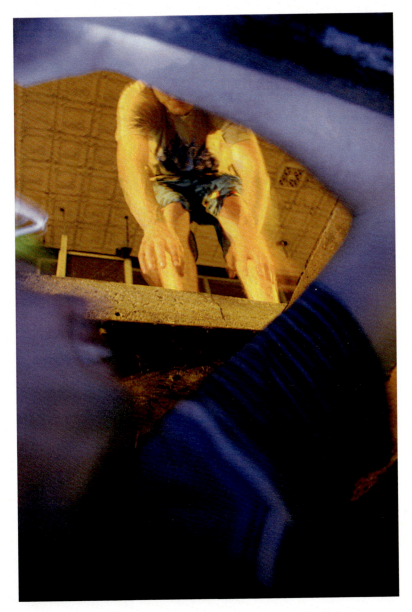

Tricksters – Emerging from underground spaces in unexpected places

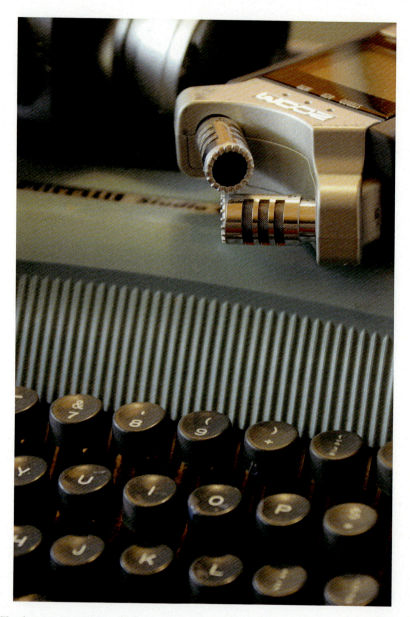

Tools – A Super 8 camera, an environmental audio-recorder, and a manual typewriter

The image presents a conundrum to research on non-representational geographies. How is it *not* representational? In a discipline so obsessed with the visual (Rose 2003), how can we regard photography as anything other than the "appropriation of the thing being photographed" (Sontag 1973, p. 2)? In my research, I have deliberately avoided the typical, 'show and tell' of research photography, opting instead to present only a small number of images together as a kind of visual interlude. In so doing, however, a whole set of different assumptions are deployed about what images 'do'. In this respect, I was inspired by Roberts (2012) recasting of research photographs as empirical hauntings that lie somewhere between the material and immaterial, the real and the virtual.

Thinking the image beyond representation is to explore different ways of seeing – including the way that seeing affects us (Berger 2008). It means opening photography up to questions of "duration, narration and movement", by bringing the image's intense and affective qualities to the fore (Bleyen 2012, p. ix). I did this in three ways in the research. The first was to photograph fast movements with a moderate exposure – this leaves a 'trace' that emphasises the temporal quality of the image (Plummer 2012). The second was the use of photomontage (Ades 1976) as a 'tool for thought'. The third was the use of stop-frame animation (Gasek 2013) to produce short segments of video, some of which were incorporated into a short film, which was later exhibited. I will consider each of these before turning, briefly, to the making of the film.

Photographs are not instantaneous. They are time exposures, which capture a distinct period of time (Szarkowski 1966). Photographs and film can only ever provide an illusion of movement, however, by recreating it as an image. Film recreates movement through a series of successive images, whereas photography captures the entire duration that unfolds before it. Setting a still camera for a medium or long exposure allows the instrument to function somewhat like a movie camera in that the shutter is held open and a series of 'shots' are superimposed on the same frame (Plummer 2012). As Plummer (2012) argues, photographs taken with long exposures trace a continuity of movement – not only extending the time of the photograph but also revealing that time in its image. For Bleyen (2012), photographs that extend or experiment with the medium can be considered as a 'minor' photography, providing a 'break' from representation. Like Deleuze's concept of 'minor literature', minor photography aims to foreground the affective and intensive qualities of the world in ways that 'stutter and stammer' (O'Sullivan 2012).

Some of my fieldwork photographs appeared static. It is in these photographs that I attempted to present something of the materials of art practice or the instruments of the research. This was done as a reversal of the traditional 'human pose' by objectifying the non-human in the form of a 'close up' (see Deleuze 1983 on affection-images). By employing 'durational photography', however, I attempted to present the affective, expressive, and relational qualities of therapeutic art making by decentring the human subject. This form of photography captures affective events – events of becoming and subjectivation. This style involves an intentional avoidance of the affection-image (i.e., close-ups of the human face) and an emphasis on bodily movement and relation. The photomontages produced in the process of this research combined stills of the non-human with durational photography in the attempt to disrupt time in a kind of *affective stammering* (O'Sullivan 2012). This presents spaces of therapeutic art making as "zones where living beings whirl around" (Deleuze and Guattari 1994, p. 173).

Stop-frame animation, or stop-motion animation, takes many different forms. Two of the most popular are clay animation and pixilation (Gasek 2013). In clay animation a puppet or clay figure with flexible parts is photographed, frame-by-frame, after slight adjustments are made to its position. When 'stitched' together, digitally, the frame-by-frame produces the semblance of smooth movement. In pixilation, a human subject poses under similar conditions. In pixilation, however, the idea is to disrupt our normal perception of human movement by producing animations that are stilted, jerky, streaky, or ethereal. Another form of stop-frame animation is brief, time-lapse photography – a form made much easier by the use of digital cameras. Cameras in time-lapse mode take photographs of a moving subject at regular intervals and at high shutter speeds. 'Stitching' these photographs together in succession creates a similar aesthetic to pixilation but speeds up time, exaggerating movement.

Two segments of stop-frame animation produced via time-lapse photography were included in the short film. The first, as previously described, depicts Swagata's ekphrastic painting of her own dance. Despite the rapid shutter speed, Swagata's movements are sometimes so fast that they leave a movement trace. The second stop-frame animation appears later in the film and demonstrates the peripheral practice of fire-setting in which drain art practitioners sometimes engage. The stop-frame here works to emphasise the sudden 'explosion' of light from within an otherwise dark space and the flickering of fire as it slowly 'dies'.

Doel and Clarke (2007) argue that "montage is at the very heart of contemporary human geography" (p. 890). This is because its process of selecting, editing, juxtaposing, and 'piecing together' of disparate images for effect deliberately privileges "politics over aesthetics and of substances over style" (p. 890). Doel and Clarke (2007) suggest that montage provides 'shocks' to content that invoke 'eventfulness', affect, materialities, disclosure, intercession, readiness, and the politics of witnessing. This is why Doel and Clarke (2007) believe that montage is the "essential gesture of nonrepresentational styles of thought and action [that] makes the Open palpable and formlessness tangible" (p. 899). Two aspects of montage, stoppage and repetition, are particularly relevant in this regard as they enable film to express the multiplicity of becoming. To stop and restart image is to interrupt its meaning, to create resistance, and to introduce 'ands' and 'buts' that sweep the viewer up into a becoming world. The viewer is 'plunged' into the montage and its own reality as it produces a semblance of a world that is produced, rather than ready-made.

Montage was a feature of neo-avant-garde film making, an art movement which reached its height in the late 1960s (Hopkins 2006). This corresponded to the advent of portable Super 8 camera. Super 8 images have a particularly diaphanous quality. Images are desaturated, emphasising the material qualities of surfaces, and the play of light and shadow. This effect is still discernable after the telecine process – the frame-by-frame transfer of film to digital data. It is difficult to focus a Super 8 camera. This temporary loss of focus is disorienting for the viewer. By incorporating a much braver array of poetic/musical ekphrasis and soundscape, alongside Super 8 footage, stop-frame animations, and still photographs, I produced a short film of 20 minutes duration (Boyd 2013). The film cuts across several variations in sound and image. This effect is enhanced further by the use of digital filters as well as manual distortion of the film by hand scraping and staining prior to the telecine process.

Two practices that had not yet featured in the ekphrastic work (but were included in poetic accounts; Boyd forthcoming) were slow art and group dance therapy. The materialities and affective qualities of these practices are borne out in the film with the aid of contrast. The combination of musical ekphrasis with avant-garde-style images creates tension. For me as the artist, this tension was greatest between the central segment of colour Super 8 against the final segment of black and white. The colour footage was shot at night, whereas the black and white was shot during the day. The colour footage is of a night-time painting session focused (almost) on the rough, frenetic, and impulsive movements that I typically make when I paint. The final segment is of Amanda Robins' slow art. As indicated in the poetic accounts, this practice is slow, gentle, and soft. The dance of light in the final segment bears this out beautifully, as does the light plucking and strumming of guitar strings. In the colour segment, the rough, jerky movements of the camera, the frequent loss of focus, and the shock of colour in the dark are complemented by the shrieking of wind instruments and the straining of a 'just' audible voice.

Although, I can only regret that the montage could not incorporate haptics, taste, or smell, the particular melding of image and sound in the montage, and the aporia this induces in the viewer, makes it an exemplary form of affective knowledge translation. Dewsbury (2009b) argues that avant-garde techniques have a special ability to emphasise experience, performance, and expression. In the short film, this is emphasised further by the cutting through of image and sound and the use of Super 8 footage. Sager-Eidt (2008) calls the melding of image and sound in this way 'film as ekphrasis' – the ekphrastic encounter being between artist and practice, viewer and form, in this case creating an ekphrastic geography capable of bringing therapeutic art making 'to life'.

CHAPTER 6

Interstices of Becoming

Abstract Seven propositions arising from the research are presented in this chapter, relating to (1) the senses, (2) space and context, (3) materiality, the non-human and the ontic, (4) attunement and fielding, (5) affective knowledge translation, (6) change and transformation, and (7) interstices of becoming.

Keywords Attunement · Fielding · Affective knowledge translation · Change and transformation · Becoming

This book details a scholarly endeavour fuelled by a blaze of post-structuralist thought. My intention with this chapter, however, is to not reference anyone or anything. It will be an unfolding of my own thought, based on theory-informed practice, and presented as a series of seven propositions.

PROPOSITION 1: THE SENSES

Sight, sound, taste, touch, and smell...together they are heightened or entrained in events of therapeutic art making. As a practitioner of subterranean graffiti, I am overwhelmed by the sonic power of the drain environment. As a dancer of the five rhythms, I am enveloped by the smell of sweaty bodies and the taste of sweat on my lips. In acts of visual art making, my eyes are saturated by vivid colour as the palette knife moves through

© The Author(s) 2017
C.P. Boyd, *Non-Representational Geographies of Therapeutic Art Making*, DOI 10.1007/978-3-319-46286-8_6

thick, sticky, and gooey substances. In a community of activist gardeners, my hands contact cool, moist soil. Someone gives me a berry straight from the bush and its freshness explodes in my mouth. Working with fibre, I encounter the material resilience of cloth or wool – at once strong and soft.

The heightening of sense is not in itself therapeutic. It becomes therapeutic as part of an ethical experience of relating to the world. This has less to do with perception and more to do with what is perceptively felt. A sensing body in relation is a synaesthetic one, enrolling all of the active senses in the encounter. It is ethical, because it is generative. A sensing body in relation is also a body in movement, with a heightened *kinaesthetic* and *proprioceptive* sense. Although I cannot help but move in relation, this movement becomes therapeutic when I become aware that I do not move in isolation. I move in relation to human and non-human 'others'.

Sensory experience *refrains* in therapeutic encounters. It is, however, a difference-producing repetition. When I move through paint with a knife, repeatedly carving, moulding, and dispersing it, I produce something new. I feel that my movements gather a creative momentum as something starts to emerge from the effort. I see it with my eyes and feel it in my hands, but I also experience it as embodied rhythm. Small, repetitive brush strokes against canvas, the hissing strokes that rush out of paint cans, the scraping of a rake over a new garden path, the casting on of a stitch followed by the casting on of another. Small, mundane movements are painstakingly repeated in minute bursts of sensation that broadcast 'the refrain'. In some instances this might soothe me, in others it might excite me, but it is always in excess of me.

In certain moments, I might experience pure sensation, or the extension of my body to the whole, sensible world. This is an experience of sensation as vibration, as *pure presence* that escapes the body. This is somewhere outside my general experience of the world – that is, beyond contemplation or a cognitive register. In these instances, the senses come together to form a unity that expresses itself in chaos. These moments are perhaps the most therapeutic of all, because they 'out run' me, leaving me behind, allowing me to 'lose' myself in the world.

PROPOSITION 2: SPACE AND CONTEXT

Spaces of therapeutic art making are temporarily acquired and co-constructed. Effectively, they are shared. When my fellow artists and I infiltrate Melbourne's system of underground drain tunnels, we do not appropriate them for our own purposes. The drain invites us in. It is our host for the evening. When I do a painting at home, my living room becomes a studio – the floor becomes the easel. A church hall on a Tuesday evening, pumping with electronic music and the co-mingling of dancers, becomes a very different therapeutic space from what it was on a Sunday. Therapeutic art making transmutes spaces into contexts that privilege embodied action in ways that 'the clinic' does not.

This is an understanding of space and context as performative. Performances always take place in concert and in relation. As spaces of co-intensive sensing, therapeutic contexts of this nature transform subjects by foregrounding the processes of life's emergence. We come to know what is outside of the mind, beyond representation, as it is experienced in the moment. Spaces of therapeutic art making are 'eventful' spaces where things happen that guide willing participants towards ethical acts of self-care and self-expression. These are intensive spaces, carved out in the service of a need to 'feel the world'.

Therapy has always been appreciated as a process but rarely as an event. We are taught to believe that the 'process' results in an outcome that was somehow 'caused'. Events of therapeutic art making, however, are singularities. It is at the border, where the virtual leaks into the actual, that transformation really takes place. As such, therapy of this kind (or perhaps any kind) is best regarded as a 'passing on' or a 'passing through'. Its processes are ones of interlocking experiences. The subject is caught up, swept up, in the event and, at the same time, diminished by it. Not lessened but distributed in agency. This means that therapeutic experiences can be non-intentional, without form or internal directedness, precognitive, and pre-reflexive.

PROPOSITION 3: MATERIALITY, THE NON-HUMAN, AND THE ONTIC

Thinking in relation to matter opens up the world to the possibilities of practice and performance. When objects are not just considered as tools to be appropriated for human use, they become expressive, and it is material expressions that make up the natural world. Freeing matter from the constraints of representation allows us to celebrate its dynamic qualities. It also promotes *transversal* modes of becoming. Elevating the status of the material world involves recognising our own materiality and emphasising the shared status of all things.

Raising the status of the non-human does not mean that human relationships do not exert a powerful influence over our 'individual' sense of well-being. It does, however, expand the notion of wellness to the more-than-human world. In so doing, it also extends what it means to *belong* by increasing our capacity to act ethically, in relation to all forms of life and non-life. It fosters an awareness of joint action and its material consequences. It decentres agency, encouraging social responsibility and corporeal sensibilities. Because the living body extends to the whole, sensible world then we are able to discover the ways in which we, as humans, contribute to a wider ecology of things – through our presence but also through our absence. If we acknowledge the 'ontic' (or the ontological status of objects as independent from our 'will') then we must also acknowledge that there are things that we can never know, because they exist outside of our experience. This radically challenges typical conceptions of being and becoming by introducing the notion of chance. We are not sovereign. The world reveals itself to us. We are not its maker. The world irrupts out of nothing, and it will continue to do so long after 'we' are gone.

Proposition 4: Attunement and Fielding

Geographical fieldwork has always involved 'going out into the world' to discover something new (with all the attendant 'sovereign' trappings that this entails). Geography is perhaps the most diverse of all academic disciplines in that geographers deploy methods across the entire breadth of programmatic research – from positivism, to constructivism, and the performative. Researching the non-representational, however, does not require prescribed methods. What it requires is the development of sensory attunement, the gathering of embodied knowledge, and techniques for translating that knowledge into forms that can be audienced.

The concept of sensory attunement is very difficult to pin down. For me, the experience of biofeedback provides a useful analogy. My first experience of biofeedback was in a clinic where I worked. A psychiatrist brought in a 'machine' so that my colleagues and I could 'play'. More recently, I was in hospital hooked up to a monitor and in my boredom, experimented with lowering my heart rate by focusing on it. Lowering one's heart rate by thinking involves an initial moment of intense focus followed by a letting go of that focus. The intense focus is aimed at the monitor, and the letting go returns across the intervening space back to the body as a 'felt' perception of bodily rhythm. It works, but I cannot explain how or why. It works every single time, albeit for a very brief moment. Presumably it involves some form of neurological feedback mechanism, but it is not experienced this way. It is experienced as attunement – an intense focus, followed by a redounding of thought across space, returning as embodied perception.

Fielding is different. Fielding is a technique for opening out perception to take in as much of the field as possible. It is the dispersal of attention. For me, it is like the experience of mindfulness meditation but even wider. In cultivating 'fielding' as a technique I needed to learn how to flatten my perception. In mindfulness meditation, I am firmly in the centre of the field with the environment circulating around me. To 'field' is to decentre oneself by inviting 'chaos' in. It's 'noisy' in that way. My perception 'escapes' my body in these moments and is given the freedom to explore geographies outside of my subject-centred understandings.

In terms of therapeutics, attunement and fielding are powerful conceptual tools for developing 'techniques of lived abstraction'. They are ways of thinking, feeling, and perceiving that treat knowledge as action and life as emergent. As such, attunement and fielding are not just a requirement for 'doing' non-representational geographies; they are transformative in and of themselves.

Proposition 5: Affective Knowledge Translation

Non-representational theory is a call to witness 'the already witnessing world'. This, however, is not knowledge for the sake of itself but knowledge for the world's sake. 'Minor' knowledges disrupt the 'will to power' of the 'major' by producing knowledges that confront the dominant social paradigm – a pattern of thinking which asserts that humans are superior to all other forms of life. Academic discourses and practices are particularly vulnerable to this paradigm by placing so much emphasis on personal authorship, rankings, impact, and esteem. Affective knowledge, however, cannot be owned. It is shared between the world and me. By trading in modes of perception that are fleeting, ephemeral, and atmospheric, non-representational theory valorises the things we come to know that are outside of our will and intention. Knowledge of this kind is an open, yet contextual, grasping – aporetic and uncertain.

Affective knowledge only 'works' in translation. Although creative practice is now a valid mode of inquiry within the academy it can only ever be partially represented in words. For the most part, the knowledges produced are non-representational – embodied in artworks or performances – and, therefore, must be audienced to be communicated. However, audiences *receive* affective knowledge in ways that cannot be predicted or ensured. From the artist's point of view, it is an attempt to convey a conceptual feeling, but it cannot be anything other than an attempt. It might succeed or it might fail, and the experience of it will be different for each person who witnesses it. Moreover, it is only ever experienced as an encounter with the potential to be re-experienced in a multitude of ways. What this means is that affective knowledge gains must be tentative – framed as propositions rather than conclusions. In so doing, they remain open. However, this is not 'weak knowledge'. The power of affective knowledge gains, and perhaps their greatest contribution to the academy, is that they *participate* in knowledge production in ways that resist foreclosure.

Proposition 6: Change and Transformation

When therapy is an event and not an outcome, change must be seen as process and transformation as an experience. Transformation is experienced in the event and is, therefore, temporal. Change takes place in relation and is, therefore, spatial. Change and transformation, in this regard, are not psychological (i.e., arising from the mind) but geographical (i.e., occurrences of space–time). They are actualisations of the potential that already exists in the world.

When we understand that the 'self' is geographically constituted, then we can accept that change and transformation cannot be engineered. They occur by chance. They are 'lines of flight'. What can be cultivated, however, is an open and sensuous disposition, an increased capacity to be affected, and the ability to construct spaces and contexts that allow 'lines of flight' to occur more easily. These are the non-striated, smooth spaces of therapeutic art making or any other ethico-aesthetic activity that creates universes of value – the kind of change and transformation that comes about from living 'minor'.

Proposition 7: Interstices of Becoming

Acts of therapeutic art making are not always gentle and peaceful. They can be violent, aggressive, exhausting, and intense. It is in these moments of affective intensity, however, that interstices of becoming are temporarily realised. Interstices of becoming create 'lures of feeling' that allow us to 'process the real', to 'wonder the world directly', and to contact the virtual. They are so very, very small, but they are also the most powerful of all spaces that involve us as humans, because they are generative – generative of change, generative of thought, and generative of ethical action (respectively, what it means to be a socially engaged artist, a philosopher, or a subtle activist). Ultimately, acts of therapeutic art making enrich lives by creating opportunities to participate ethically in the world in a manner that respects life, because 'I' (finally) come to understand that 'my life is not mine'.

REFERENCES

Abram, D. (1996). *The spell of the sensuous: Perception and language in a more-than-human world*. New York: Vintage Books.

Abram, D. (2010). *Becoming animal: An earthly cosmology*. New York: Vintage Books.

Ades, D. (1976). *Photomontage*. London: Thames and Hudson.

Adey, P., Brayer, L., Masson, D., Murphy, P., Simpson, P., & Tixier, N. (2013). *Pour votre tranquillité*: Ambiance, atmosphere, and surveillance. *Geoforum, 49*, 209–309.

Anderson, B. (2006). Becoming and being hopeful: Towards a theory of affect. *Environment and Planning D: Society and Space, 24*, 733–752.

Anderson, B. (2009). Affective atmospheres. *Emotion, Space and Society, 2*, 77–81.

Anderson, B. (2014). *Encountering affect: Capacities, apparatuses, conditions*. Farnham: Ashgate.

Anderson, B., & Harrison, P. (2010). The promise of non-representational theories. In B. Anderson & P. Harrison, *Taking-place: Non-representational theories and human geography*. London: Ashgate.

Anderson, B., & Wylie, J. (2009). On geography and materiality. *Environment and Planning A, 41*, 318–335.

Anonymous (2012). *Entries in the visitors' book: Non-representational geographies of therapeutic art making exhibition*. University of Melbourne, 10 December.

Ash, J. (2013a). Rethinking affective atmospheres: Technology, perturbation and space times of the non-human'. *Geoforum, 49*, 20–28.

Ash, J. (2013b). Technologies of captivation: Videogames and the attunement of affect. *Body and Society, 19*, 27–35.

Ash, J., & Simpson, P. (2014). Geography and post-phenomenology. *Progress in Human Geography*. doi:10.1177/0309132514544806.

© The Author(s) 2017
C.P. Boyd, *Non-Representational Geographies of Therapeutic Art Making*, DOI 10.1007/978-3-319-46286-8

100 REFERENCES

Bachelard, G. (1994). *The poetics of space.* (trans: Maria Jolas). Boston: Beacon.

Bachelard, G. (2005). *On poetic imagination and reverie.* (trans: Colette Gaudin). Putnam: Spring.

Barad, K. (2007). *Meeting the universe halfway: Quantum physics and the entanglement of matter and meaning.* Durham: Duke University Press.

Barrett, E. (2010). The exegesis as meme. In E. Barrett & B. Bolt (eds.), *Practice as research: Approaches to creative arts enquiry.* London: I.B. Tauris.

Barrett, E., & Bolt, B. (2013). *Carnal knowledge: Towards a 'new materialism' through the arts.* London: I.B. Tauris.

Bennett, J. (2001). *The enchantment of modern life: Attachments, crossings, and ethics.* Princeton: Princeton University Press.

Bennett, J. (2010). *Vibrant matter: A political ecology of things.* Durham: Duke University Press.

Berger, J. (2008). *Ways of seeing.* London: Penguin Books.

Bergson, H. (2004). *Matter and memory.* (trans: Nancy Marget Paul and W. Scott Palmer). Mineola: Dover.

Bertelson, L. (2013). Francesca Woodman: Becoming-woman, becoming-imperceptible, becoming-a-subject-in-wonder. *Performance Paradigm: A Journal of Performance and Contemporary Culture, 9,* 5.

Bissell, D. (2009). Obdurant pains, transient intensities: Affect and the chronically pained body. *Environment and Planning A,* 41, 911–928.

Bissell, D. (2010). Passenger mobilities: Affective atmospheres and the sociality of public transport. *Environment and Planning D: Society and Space, 28,* 270–289.

Bissell, D. (2012). Agitating the powers of habit: Towards a volatile politics of thought. *Theory and Event, 15.* doi:10.1353/tae.2012.0000.

Bissell, D., & Fuller, G. (2009). Stillness unbound. In D. Bissell & G. Fuller (eds.), *Stillness in a mobile world.* Abingdon: Routledge.

Blackman, L. (2008). *The body: The key concepts.* Oxford: Berg.

Blackman, L. (2012). *Immaterial bodies: Affect, embodiment, mediation.* London: Sage.

Bleyen, M. (2012). Introduction. In M. Bleyen (ed.), *Minor photography: Connecting Deleuze and Guattari to photography theory.* Leuven: Leuven University Press.

Bolt, B. (2007). Material thinking and the agency of matter. *Studies in Material Thinking, 1,* online.

Bolt, B. (2010). The magic is in the handling. In E. Barrett & B. Bolt (eds.), *Practice as research: Approaches to creative arts enquiry.* London: I.B. Tauris.

Bolt, B. (2011). *Heidegger Reframed.* London: I.B. Tauris.

Bolter, J.D. (2001). *Writing space: Computers, hypertext, and the remediation of print.* New York: Routledge.

REFERENCES 101

Bondi, L. (2005). Making connections and thinking through emotions: Between geography and psychotherapy. *Transactions of the Institute of British Geographers*, 30, 433–448.

Bondi, L., & Davidson, J. (2011). Lost in translation. *Transactions of the British Institute of Geographers*, 36, 595–598.

Bowden, S. (2011). *The priority of events: Deleuze's logic of sense.* Edinburgh: Edinburgh University Press.

Boyd, C.P. (2013). *Sound as ekphrasis: Affective responses to therapeutic art-making* [videorecording, 19 mins]. Available at: https://vimeo.com/56185606.

Boyd, C.P. (forthcoming). Forces, flows, and vital materialisms in therapeutic art making: A poetic account of contemporary geographical fieldwork. Under review with. *ACME: An International Journal for Critical Geographies*.

Braidotti, R. (2006). *Transpositions: On nomadic ethics.* Cambridge: Polity.

Braidotti, R. (2011a). *Nomadic subjects: Embodiment and sexual difference in contemporary feminist theory.* New York: Columbia University Press.

Braidotti, R. (2011b). *Nomadic theory: The portable Rosi Braidotti.* New York: Columbia University Press.

Braidotti, R. (2013). *The posthuman.* Cambridge: Polity.

Brennan, T. (2004). *The transmission of affect.* Ithaca: Cornell University Press.

Bruhn, S. (2000). *Musical ekphrasis: Composers responding to poetry and painting.* Hillsdale: Pendragon.

Bryant, L., Srnicek, N. & Harman, G. (2011). *The speculative turn: Continental materialism and realism.* Melbourne: re.press

Buchanan, I. (2013). Schizoanalysis: An incomplete project. In Dillet Benoît, Iain Mackenzie & Robert Porter (eds.), *The Edinburgh companion to poststructuralism.* Edinburgh: Edinburgh University Press.

Bull, M., & Back, L. (2003). *The auditory culture reader.* Oxford: Berg.

Butler, J. (1993). *Bodies that matter: On the discursive limits of "sex".* New York: Routledge.

Carman, T. (2008). Between empiricism and intellectualism. In R. Diprose & J. Reynolds (eds.), *Merleau-Ponty: Key concepts.* Stocksfield: Acumen.

Clough, P. (2007). *The affective turn: Theorizing the social.* (With Jean Halley). Durham: Duke University Press.

Colebrook, C. (2005). Actuality. In Adrian Parr (ed.), *The Deleuze dictionary.* New York: Columbia University Press.

Collins, L. (2014). *Making sense: Art practice and transformative therapeutics.* London: Bloomsbury.

Colls, R. (2012). Feminism, bodily difference and non-representational geographies. *Transactions of the Institute of British Geographers*, 37, 430–445.

Conradson, D. & Latham, A. (2007). The affective possibilities of London: Antipodean transnationals and the overseas experience. *Mobilities*, 2, 231–254.

102 REFERENCES

Couclelis, H. (1999). Space, time, geography. In P. Longley, M. Goodchild, D. Maguire, & D. Rhind (eds.), *Geographical information systems: Principles, techniques, management, and applications*, Vol. 1. New York: Wiley.

Crawford, N. (2013). *Theology as improvisation: A study in the musical nature of theological thinking*. Leiden: Brill.

Cregan, K. (2006). *The sociology of the body: Mapping the abstraction of embodiment*. London: Sage.

Crouch, D. (2003). Spacing, performance and becoming: The tangle of the mundane. *Environment and Planning A, 35,* 1945–1960.

Crouch, D. (2010). *Flirting with space: Journeys and creativity*. Farnham: Ashgate.

Damasio, A. (2000). *The feeling of what happens: Body and emotion in the making of consciousness*. Orlando: Harcourt.

Darwin, C. (1859). *On the origin or species by means of natural selection or the preservation of favoured races in the struggle for life*. London: John Murray, Albemarle Street.

De Certeau, M. (1984). *The practice of everyday life*. (trans: Steven Rendall). Berkeley: University of California Press.

Dean, R.T. (1989). *Creative improvisation: Jazz, contemporary music and beyond*. Milton Keynes: Open University Press.

DeFanti, T., Grafton, A., Levy, T.E., Manovich, L., & Rockwood, A. (2015). *Quantitative methods in the humanities and social sciences*. London: Springer.

DeLanda, M. (2005). Space: Extensive and intensive, actual and virtual. In I. Buchanan & G. Lambert (eds.), *Deleuze and space*. Edinburgh: Edinburgh University Press.

Deleuze, G. (1983). *Cinema 1: The movement-image*. (trans: Hugh Tomlinson and Barbara Habberjam). Minneapolis: University of Minnesota Press.

Deleuze, G. (1990). *The logic of sense*. (trans: Mark Lester with Charles Stivale, Edited by Constantin V. Boundas). New York: Columbia University Press.

Deleuze, G. (1993). *The fold: Leibniz and the Baroque*. (trans: Tom Conley). Minneapolis: University of Minnesota Press.

Deleuze, G. (1994). *Difference and repetition*. (trans: Paul Patton). New York: Columbia University Press.

Deleuze, G. (2000). *Proust and signs: The complete text*. (trans: Richard Howard). Minneapolis: University of Minnesota Press.

Deleuze, G., & Guattari, F. (1987). *A thousand plateaus: Capitalism and schizophrenia*. (trans: Brian Massumi). Minneapolis: University of Minnesota Press.

Deleuze, G., & Guattari, F. (1994). *What is philosophy?* (trans: Hugh Tomlinson and Graham Burchell). New York: Columbia University Press.

Deleuze, G., & Parnet, C. (1987). *Dialogues*. (trans: Hugh Tomlinson and Barbara Habberjam). New York: Columbia University Press.

REFERENCES 103

Destrual, P. (1998). Bachelard, et l'imaginaire de l'espace nervalien selon Richard et Poulet. *Revue Romane, 33*, 107–125.

Dewsbury, J.-D., Harrison, P., Rose, M. and Wylie, J. (2002). Enacting geographies. *Geoforum, 33*, 437–440.

Dewsbury, J.-D. (2003). Witnessing space: 'Knowing without contemplation'. *Environment and Planning A, 35*, 1907–1932.

Dewsbury, J.-D. (2009a). Performative, non-representational, and affect-based research: Seven injunctions. In D. DeLyser, S. Herbert, S. Aitken, M. Crang, & L. McDowell (eds.), *The SAGE handbook of qualitative geography*. London: Sage.

Dewsbury, J.-D. (2009b). Avant-garde/avant-garde geographies. In R. Kitchen & N. Thrift (eds.), *International encyclopedia of human geography*. London: Elsevier.

Dewsbury, J.-D. (2010). Language and the event: The unthought of appearing worlds. In B. Anderson & P. Harrison (eds.), *Taking place: Non-representational theories and geography*. Farnham: Ashgate.

Dewsbury, J.-D. (2012). Affective habit ecologies: Material dispositions and immanent inhabitations. *Performance Research: A Journal of the Performing Arts, 17*, 74–82.

Dewsbury, J.-D., & Thrift, N. (2005). 'Genesis eternal': After Paul Klee. In I. Buchanan & G. Lambert (eds.), *Deleuze and space*. Edinburgh: Edinburgh University Press.

Dieter, M. (2013). New materialism and non-humanisation: An interview with Jussi Parikka In M. Kasprzak (curator) *Blowup–Speculative Realities*. Rotterdam: The Netherlands.

Dixon, D.P., & Straughan, E.R. (2010). Geographies of touch/touched by geography. *Geography Compass, 4/5*, 449–459.

Doel, M.A. (2010). Representation and difference. In B. Anderson & P. Harrison, *Taking-place: Non-representational theories and human geography*. London: Ashgate.

Doel, M.A., & Clarke, D.B. (2007). Afterimages. *Environment and Planning D: Society and Space, 25*, 890–910.

Dolphijn, R., & Van Der Tuin, I. (2012). *New materialism: Interviews and cartographies*. Ann Arbor: Open University Press.

Drobnick, J. (2006). *The smell culture reader*. Oxford: Berg.

Duffy, M., Waitt, G., Gorman-Murray, A., & Gibson, C. (2011). Bodily rhythms: Corporeal capacities to engage with festival spaces. *Emotion, Space and Society, 4*, 17–24.

Duffy, S. (2012). The question of Deleuze's neo-Leibnizianism. In R. Braidotti & P. Pisters (eds.), *Revisiting normativity with Deleuze*. Bloomsbury: London.

Durant, A. (1989). Improvisation in the political economy of music. In C. Norris (ed.), *Music and the politics of culture*. New York: St Martin's Press.

104 REFERENCES

Evens, A. (2002). Sound Ideas. In B. Massumi (ed.), *A shock to thought: Expression after Deleuze and Guattari*. New York: Routledge.

Ferrington, G. (1994). Audio design: Creating multisensory images for the mind. *Journal of Visual Literacy, 14*, 61–67.

Flick, U. (2009). *An introduction to qualitative research*. London: Sage.

Ford, L.S. (1984). *The emergence of Whitehead's metaphysics: 1925–1929*. New York: State University of New York Press.

Foucault, M. (1971). *The order of things: An archeology of the human sciences*. New York: Pantheon Books.

Foucault, M. (1973). *The birth of the clinic: An archaeology of medical perception*. New York: Pantheon.

Frisina, W.G. (2002). *The unity of knowledge and action: Toward a nonrepresentational theory of knowledge*. New York: State University of New York Press.

Gallagher, M. (2014). Sounding ruins: Reflections on the production of an 'audio drift'. *Cultural Geographies, 21*, 1–19.

Gallagher, M. (2015). Field recording and the sounding of spaces. *Environment and Planning D: Society and Space, 33*, 560–576.

Gallagher, M., & Prior, J. (2014). Sonic geographies: Exploring phonographic methods. *Progress in Human Geography, 38*, 267–284.

Gandelman, C. (1991). *Reading pictures, viewing texts*. Bloomington: Indiana University Press.

Garrett, B.L. (2013). *Explore everything: Place-hacking the city*. London: Verso.

Gasek, T. (2013). *Frame-by-frame stop motion: The guide to non-traditional animation techniques*. New York: Focal Press.

Genosko, G. (2002). *Félix Guattari: An abberant introduction*. London: Continuum.

Gilleard, C., & Higgs, P. (2013). *Ageing, corporeality and embodiment*. London: Anthem.

Goddard, S. (2010). A correspondence between practices. In E. Barrett & B. Bolt (eds.), *Practice as research: Approaches to creative arts enquiry*. London: I.B. Tauris.

Grech, J. (2006). Practice-led research and scientific knowledge. *Media International Australia incorporating Culture and Policy, 118*, 34–42.

Grene, M. (1993). The primacy of the ecological self. In U. Neisser (ed.), *The perceived self: Ecological and interpersonal sources of self-knowledge*. Cambridge: Cambridge University Press.

Grosz, E. (1994). *Volatile bodies: Towards a corporeal feminism*. Bloomington: Indiana University Press.

Grosz, E. (1995). *Space, time, perversion: Essays on the politics of bodies*. New York: Routledge.

Grosz, E. (2005). Bergson, Deleuze and the becoming of unbecoming. *Parallax, 11*, 4–13.

REFERENCES 105

Grosz, E. (2008). *Chaos, territory, art: Deleuze and the framing of the earth.* New York: Columbia University Press.

Grosz, E. (2013). Habit today: Ravaisson, Bergson, Deleuze and us. *Body and Society, 19,* 217–239.

Guattari, F. (1989). The three ecologies. (Tran: Chris Turner). *New formations, 8,* 131–147.

Guattari, F. (1995). *Chaosmosis: An ethico-aesthetic paradigm* (Tran: Paul Bains and Justin Pefanis). Bloomington: Indiana University Press.

Guattari, F. (1996). *The Guattari reader: Pierre-Félix Guattari,* (edited by Gary Genosko). Oxford: Blackwell.

Guattari, F. (2013). *Schizoanalytic cartographies.* London: Bloomsbury.

Gumbrecht, H. G. (2004). *The production of presence: What meaning cannot convey.* Redwood City: Stanford University Press.

Hardy, T., & Danvers, J. (2006). The knowing body: Art as an integrative system of knowledge. In T. Hardy (ed.), *Art education in a postmodern world.* Bristol: Intellect.

Harman, G. (2002). *Tool-being: Heidegger and the metaphysics of objects.* Chicago: Open Court.

Harman, G. (2012). The Third Table/Der dritte Tisch: 100 Notes–100 thoughts/100 Notizen–100 Gedanken no. 85. *dOCUMENTA (13).* Kassel: Erschienen im Hatje Cantz.

Harman, G. (2013). The current state of speculative realism. *Speculations: A Journal of Speculative Realism, IV,* 22–28.

Harrison, P. (2007). "*How shall I say it ...?*" Relating the nonrelational. *Environment and Planning A, 39,* 590–608.

Haseman, B. (2006). A manifesto for performative research. *Media International Australia incorporating Culture and Policy, 118,* 98–106.

Haseman, B. (2010). Rupture and recognition: Identifying the performative research paradigm. In E. Barrett & B. Bolt (eds.), *Practice as research: Approaches to creative arts enquiry.* London: I.B. Tauris.

Haseman, B., & Mafe, D. (2009). Acquiring know-how: Research training for practice-led researchers. In H. Smith & R.T. Dean (eds.), *Practice-led research, research-led practice in the creative arts.* Edinburgh: Edinburgh University Press.

Hawkins, H. (2014). *For creative geographies: Geography, visual arts and the making of worlds.* New York: Routledge.

Hayes, L., Bach, P.A., & Boyd, C.P. (2010). Psychological treatment for adolescent depression: Perspectives on the past, present, and future. *Behaviour Change, 27,* 1–18.

Heidegger, M. (1962). *Being and time.* (trans: John Macquarrie and Edward Robinson). New York: Harper and Row.

Hopkins, D. (2006). *Neo-avant-garde.* Amsterdam: Rodopi.

106 REFERENCES

Hosinski, T.E. (1993). *Stubborn fact and creative advance: An introduction to the metaphysics of Alfred North Whitehead.* Lanham: Rowman and Littlefield.

Idhe, D. (2003). Auditory imagination. In M. Bull & L. Back (eds.), *The auditory culture reader.* New York: Berg.

Irigaray, L. (1993). *An ethics of sexual difference.* (trans: Carolyn Burke and Gillian C. Gill). Ithaca: Cornell University Press.

James, I. (2012). *The new French philosophy.* Cambridge: Polity.

Jellis, T. (2014). Guattari, Felix 2012 Schizoanalytic Cartographies, reviewed by Thomas Jellis. *Society and Space Open Journal.* (posted 19 July).

Kalmanowitz, D. (2013). On the seam: Fiction as truth–what can art do? In S. McNiff (ed.), *Art as research: Opportunities and challenges.* Bristol: Intellect.

Kennedy, D. (2012). *The ekphrastic encounter in contemporary British poetry and elsewhere.* Farnham: Ashgate.

King, S. (2010). *On writing: A memoir of the craft.* New York: Scribner.

Klages, M. (2012). *Key terms in literary theory.* London: Continuum.

Knill, P.J., Levine, E.G., & Levine, S.K. (2005). *Principles and practice of expressive arts therapy: Toward a therapeutic aesthetics.* London: Jessica Kinsley Publications.

Kraftl, P. (2013). *Geographies of alternative education.* Bristol: Polity.

Krieger, M. (1992). *Ekphrasis: The illusion of the natural sign.* Baltimore: John Hopkins University Press.

Langer, M.M. (1989). *Merleau-Ponty's phenomenology of perception: A guide and commentary.* Houndmills: Macmillan.

Latour, B. (2007). *Reassembling the social: An introduction to actor-network-theory.* Oxford: Oxford University Press.

Lauriault, T.P., & Lindgaard, G. (2004). Scented cybercartography: Exploring possibilities. *Cartographica, 14,* 73–91.

Laurier, E., & Philo, C. (2006). Possible geographies: A passing encounter in a café. *Area, 38,* 353–363.

Lawlor, L. (2003). *Thinking through French philosophy.* Bloomington: Indiana University Press.

Lawlor, L. (2012). Phenomenology and metaphysics, and chaos: On the fragility of the event in Deleuze. In Daniel W. Smith & Henry Somers-Hall (eds.), *The Cambridge companion to Deleuze.* Cambridge: Cambridge University Press.

Lefebvre, H. (1991). *The production of space.* (trans: Donald Nicholson-Smith). Oxford: Blackwell.

Lincoln, Y.S., & Denzin, N.K. (2003). *Turning points in qualitative research: Tying knots in a handkerchief.* Walnut Creek: Altamira Press.

Lorimer, H. (2005). Cultural geography: The busyness of being 'more-than-representational'. *Progress in Human Geography, 29,* 83–94.

REFERENCES 107

Lorimer, H. (2010). Caught in the nick of time: Archives and fieldwork. In D. DeLyser, S. Herbert, S. Aitken, M. Crang, & L. McDowell (eds.), *The SAGE handbook of qualitative geography*. London: Sage.

Lorimer, H., & Parr, H. (2014). Excursions–telling stories and journeys. *Cultural Geographies, 21*, 543–547.

Loveland, K. (1993). Autism, affordances, and the self. In U. Neisser (ed.), *The perceived self: Ecological and interpersonal sources of self-knowledge*. Cambridge: Cambridge University Press.

Lynch, M. (2000). Against reflexivity as an academic virtue and source of privileged knowledge. *Theory, Culture, Society, 17*, 26–56.

Mackinlay, S. (2010). *Interpreting excess: Jean-Luc Marion, saturated phenomena, and hermeneutics*. New York: Fordham University Press.

Malabou, C. (2004). *The Heidegger change: On the fantastic in philosophy*. (trans: Peter Skafish). Albany: State University of New York Press.

Malabou, C. (2008). *What should we do with our brains?* (trans: Sebastian Rand). New York: Fordham University Press.

Manning, E. (2007). *Politics of touch: Sense, movement, sovereignty*. Minneapolis: University of Minnesota Press.

Manning, E. (2009). *Relationscapes: Movement, art, philosophy*. Cambridge: The MIT Press.

Manning, E. (2013). *Always more than one: Individuation's dance*. Durham: Duke University Press.

Manning, E. (2014). Wondering the world directly – Or, how movement outruns the subject. *Body and Society, 20*, 162–188.

Manning, E., & Massumi, B. (2014). *Thought in the act: Passages in the ecology of experience*. Minneapolis: University of Minnesota Press.

Marion, J.-L. (1998). *Reduction and givenness: Investigations of Husserl, Heidegger, and phenomenology*. (trans: Thomas A. Carlson) Evanston: Northwestern University Press.

Marion, J.-L. (2002). *Being given: Towards a phenomenology of givenness*. (trans: Jeffrey L. Kosky). Stanford: Stanford University Press.

Marion, J.-L. (2004). *The crossing of the visible*. (trans: James K.A. Smith). Stanford: Stanford University Press.

Marstaller, L. (2009). Towards a Whiteheadian neurophenomenology. *Concrescence: The Australasian Journal of Process Thought, 10*, 57–66.

Massey, D. (2005). *For space*. London: Sage.

Massumi, B. (1995). The autonomy of affect. *Cultural Critique, 31*, 83–109.

Massumi, B. (1996). Becoming-deleuzian. *Environment and Planning D: Society and Space, 14*, 395–406.

Massumi, B. (1997). The autonomy of affect. In P. Patton (ed.), *Deleuze: A critical eader*. Oxford: Blackwell.

108   REFERENCES

Massumi, B. (2002). *Parables for the virtual: Movement, affect, sensation*. Durham: Duke University Press.

Massumi, B. (2009). "Technical Mentality" revisited: Brian Massumi on Gilbert Simondon with Arne de Boever, Alex Murray and Job Roffe. *Parrhesia: A Journal of Critical Philosophy, 7*, 36–45.

Massumi, B. (2011). *Semblance and event: Arts of experience, politics of expression*. Cambridge: MIT Press.

Maturana, H. R. (2011). Ultrastability … autopoiesis? Reflective response to Tom Froese and John Stewart. *Cybernetics and Human Knowing, 18*, 143–152.

McCormack, D.P. (2002). A paper with an interest in rhythm. *Geoforum, 33*, 469–485.

McCormack, D.P. (2003). An event of geographical ethics in spaces of affect. *Transactions of the Institute of British Geographers, 28*, 488–507.

McCormack, D.P. (2005). Diagramming practice and performance. *Environment and Planning D: Society and Space, 23*, 119–147.

McCormack, D.P. (2006). For the love of pipes and cables: A response to Deborah Thien. *Area, 38*, 330–332.

McCormack, D.P. (2008a). Geographies for moving bodies: Thinking, dancing, spaces. *Geography Compass, 2*, 1822–1836.

McCormack, D.P. (2008b). Thinking-spaces for research-creation. *Inflexions, 1(1)*, 1–16.

McCormack, D.P. (2014). *Refrains for moving bodies: Experience and experiment in affective spaces*. Durham: Duke University Press.

McCosh, L. (2013). The sublime: Process and mediation. In E. Barrett & B. Bolt (eds.), *Carnal Knowledge: towards a 'New Materialism' through the arts*. London: I.B. Tauris.

McDonald, N. (2001). *The graffiti subculture: Youth, masculinity and identity in London and New York*. New York: Palgrave McMillan.

McPherson, H. (2010). Non-representational approaches to body-landscape relations. *Geography Compass, 4*, 1–13.

Meillassoux, Q. (2007). Potentiality and virtuality. *Collapse II*, 55–81.

Meillassoux, Q. (2009). *After finitude: An essay on the necessity of contingency*. (trans: Ray Brassier). London: Continuum.

Merleau-Ponty, M. (1962). *Phenomenology of perception*. (trans: Colin Smith). London: Routledge.

Merleau-Ponty, M. (1964). Eye and mind (trans: Carleton Dallery) In James M. Edie (ed.), *The primacy of perception and other essays*. Evanstone: Northwestern University Press.

Merriman, P., Jones, M., Olsson, G., Sheppard, E., Thrift, N. Tuan, Y.-F. (2012). Space and spatiality in theory. *Dialogues in Human Geography, 2*, 3–22.

Mesle, C.R. (2008). *Process-relational philosophy: An introduction to Alfred North Whitehead*. West Conshohocken: Templeton Foundation Press.

REFERENCES 109

Meyer, S. (2005). Introduction. *Configurations, 13*, 1–33.

Morris, D. (2004). *The sense of space*. Albany: State University of New York Press.

Murdoch, J. (2006). *Post-structuralist geography: A guide to relational space*. London: Sage.

Nancy, J.-L. (1993). *The birth to presence*. (trans: Brian Holmes and others). Stanford: Stanford University Press.

Nancy, J.-L. (2000). *Being singular plural*. (trans: Robert D. Richardson and Anne E. O'Bryne). Stanford: Stanford University Press.

Nancy, J.-L. (2007). *Listening*. (trans: Charlotte Mandell). New York: Fordham University Press.

Nelson, R. (2013). *Practice as research in the arts: Principles, protocols, pedagogies, resistances*. London: Palgrave Macmillan.

Nørrentranders, T. (1998). *The user illusion: Cutting consciousness down to size*. New York: Viking.

O'Sullivan, S. (2001). The aesthetics of affect: Thinking art beyond representation. *Angelaki, 6*, 125–134.

O'Sullivan, S. (2005). Notes towards a minor art practice. *Drain: Journal of Contemporary Art and Culture, 5* (online). Available at URL: http://www.drainmag.com.

O'Sullivan, S. (2006). Pragmatics for the production of subjectivity: time for probe-heads. *Journal for Cultural Research, 10*, 309–322.

O'Sullivan, S. (2007). *Academy: The production of subjectivity*. Available at URL: http://summit.kein.org/node/240.

O'Sullivan, S. (2010). Guattari's aesthetic paradigm: From the folding of the finite/infinite relation to schizoanalytic metamodelisation. *Deleuze Studies, 4(2)*, 256–286.

O'Sullivan, S. (2012). From stuttering and stammering to the diagram: Towards a minor art practice. In M. Bleyen (ed.), *Minor photography: Connecting Deleuze and Guattari to photography theory*. Leuven: Leuven University Press.

O'Sullivan, S., & Stahl, O. (2006). Contours and case studies for a dissenting subjectivity (or, how to live creatively in a fearful world). *Angelaki, 11*, 147–156.

Paterson, M. (2009). Haptic geographies: Ethnography, haptic knowledges and sensuous dispositions. *Progress in Human Geography, 33*, 766–788.

Paterson, M., & Dodge, M. (2012). *Touching space, placing touch*. Farnham: Ashgate.

Plummer, L. (2012). Photography and time duration: Time exposure and time-image. *Rhizomes, 23*, (online), n.p.

Priest, E. (2013). Felt as thought (or, musical abstraction and the semblance of affect). In M. Thompson & I. Biddle (eds.), *Sound, Music, Affect: Theorising Sonic Experience*. Bloomsbury: London.

Probyn, E. (2010). Writing shame. In M. Gregg & G. Seigworth (eds.), *The affect theory reader*. Durham: Duke University Press.

110 REFERENCES

Protevi, P. (2009). *Political affect: Connecting the social and the somatic.* Minneapolis: University of Minnesota Press.

Pylyshyn, Z.W. (2007). *Things and places: How the mind connects with the world.* Cambridge: MIT Press.

Rabinow, P. (1986). Representations are social facts: Modernity and post-modernity in anthropology. In J. Clifford & G.E. Marcus (eds.), *Writing culture: The poetics and politics of ethnography.* Berkeley: University of California Press.

Ravaisson, F. (2008). *Of habit.* (trans: Clare Carlisle and Mark Sinclair). London: Continuum.

Reason, M. (2010). Watching dance, drawing the experience and visual knowledge. *Forum for Modern Language Studies, 46,* 391–414.

Reason, M. (2012). Writing the embodied experience: Ekphrastic and creative writing as audience research. *Critical Stages, 7,* (online), n.p.

Reeves, K. in T. Dean (2013). *FILM.* Melbourne: Australian Centre for Contemporary Art.

Reynolds, R. (2009). *Transversal subjects: From Montaigne to Deleuze after Derrida.* Houndmills: Palgrave Macmillan.

Roberts, E. (2012). Geography and the visual image: A hauntological approach. *Progress in Human Geography, 37,* 386–402.

Robinson, K. (2010). Back to life: Deleuze, Whitehead and process. *Deleuze Studies, 4,* 120–133.

Rodaway, P. (1994). *Sensuous geographies: Body, sense and place.* Abingdon: Routledge.

Roelvink, G. (2010). Collective action and the politics of affect. *Emotion, Space and Society, 3,* 111–118.

Rorty, R. (1979). *Philosophy and the mirror of nature.* Princeton: Princeton University Press.

Rose, G. (2003). On the need to ask how, exactly, is geography "visual"?. *Antipode, 35,* 212–221.

Rose, N. (1996). Identity, geneology, history. In S. Hall & P. Du Gay (eds.), *Questions of cultural identity.* London: Sage.

Roth, G. (1998). *Maps to ecstasy: A healing journey for the untamed spirit.* Novato: Nataraj.

Russon, J. (1994). Embodiment and responsibility: Merleau-Ponty and the ontology of nature. *Man* (sic) *and World, 27,* 291–308.

Sager-Eidt, L.M. (2008). *Writing and filming the painting: Ekphrasis in literature and film.* London: Rodopi.

Schmid, C. (2008). Henri Lefebvre's theory of the production of space (trans: Bandulasena Goonewardena). In K. Goonewardena, S. Kipfer, R. Milgram, & C. Schmid (eds.), *Space, difference, everyday life: Reading Henri Lefebvre.* New York: Routledge.

Schrag, C.O. (1994). Transversal rationality. In T.J. Stapleton (ed.), *The question of hermeneutics*. Dordrecht: Kluwer.

Schrag, C.O. (2010). *Doing philosophy with others: Conversations, reminiscences, and reflections*. Pittsburg: Duquesne University Press.

Schroeder, F. (2015). Bringing practice closer to research – seeking integrity, sincerity and authenticity. *International Journal of Education Through Art*, *11*, 343–354.

Sedgwick, E.K. (2003). *Touching feeling: Affect, pedagogy, performativity*. Durham: Duke University Press.

Seigworth, G. (2003). Fashioning a stave, or, singing life. In J. Slack & L. Grossberg (eds.), *Animations (of Deleuze and Guattari)*. New York: Peter Lang.

Seigworth, G., & Gregg, M. (2010). Introduction. In M. Gregg & G. Seigworth (eds.), *The affect theory reader*. Durham: Duke University Press.

Serres, M. (2008). *The five senses: A philosophy of mingled bodies* (I). (trans: Margaret Sankey and Peter Cowley). London: Continuum.

Shaviro, S. (2012). *Without criteria: Kant, Whitehead, Deleuze, and Aesthetics*. Cambridge: The MIT Press.

Shipp, H. (1922). *The new art: A study of the principles of non-representational art and their application in the work of Lawrence Atkinson*. London: Cecil Palmer.

Simondon, G. (2009). Technical mentality. (trans: Arne de Boever). *Parrhesia: A Journal of Critical Philosophy*, *7*, 7–27.

Simonsen, K. (2010). Encounter O/other bodies: Practice, emotion and ethics. In B. Anderson & P. Harrison, *Taking-place: Non-representational theories and human geography*. London: Ashgate.

Simpson, P. (2009). Falling on deaf ears: A post-phenomenology of sonorous presence. *Environment and Planning A*, *41*, 2556–2575.

Simpson, P. (2011). Street performance and the city: Public space, sociality, and intervening in the everyday. *Space and Culture*, *14*, 415–430.

Smith, D. & Protevi, J. (2013). Gilles Deleuze. In Edward N. Salta (ed.), *The Stanford Encyclopedia of Philosophy*. Available from URL:: http://plato.stanford.edu/archives/spr2013/entries/deleuze/.

Smith, H., & Dean, R.T. (2009). Practice-led research, research-led practice – towards the iterative cyclic web. In H. Smith & R.T. Dean (eds.), *Practice-led research, research-led practice in the creative arts*. Edinburgh: Edinburgh University Press.

Smith, S.J. (2000). Performing the (sound)world. *Environment and Planning D: Society and Space*, *18*, 615–637.

Soja, E.W. (1996). *Thirdspace*. Oxford: Blackwell.

Sontag, S. (1964). Against interpretation. *Evergreen*, *8*, 76–80.

Sontag, S. (1973). *On photography*. New York: Rosetta Books.

112 REFERENCES

Spinney, J. (2009). Cycling the city: Movement, meaning and method. *Geography Compass, 3*, 817–835.

Spinoza, B. (2011). *Ethics.* (trans: W. H. White and Revised by A.H. Stirling]. Ware: Wordsworth.

Stengers, I. (2011). *Thinking with Whitehead: A free and wild creation of concepts.* (trans: Michael Chase). Cambridge: Harvard University Press.

Stewart, K. (2007). *Ordinary affects.* Durham: Duke University Press.

Stoller, S. (2005). Phenomenology and the poststructural critique of experience. *International Journal of Philosophical Studies, 17*, 707–737.

Sullivan, G. (2006). Research acts in art practice. *Studies in Art Education, 48*, 19–35.

Szarkowski, J. (1966). *The photographer's eye.* New York: Museum of Modern Art.

Tambornino, J. (2002). *The corporeal turn: Passion, necessity, politics.* Lanham: Rowman & Littlefield.

Tauber, Z. (2006). Aesthetic education for morality: Schiller and Kant. *The Journal of Aesthetic Education, 40*, 22–47.

Taylor, C. (1989). *Sources of the self: The making of modern identity.* Cambridge: Harvard University Press.

Thien, D. (2005). After or beyond feeling? A consideration of affect and emotion in geography. *Area, 37*, 450–454.

Thompson, M., & Biddle, I. (2013). *Sound, music, affect: Theorizing sonic experience.* London: Bloomsbury.

Thompson, N. (2012). *Living as form: Socially engaged art from 1991–2011.* Cambridge: MIT Press.

Thrift, N. (2000). Afterwords. *Environment and Planning D, 18*, 213–255.

Thrift, N. (2008a). *Non-representational theory: Space, politics, affect.* Abingdon: Routledge.

Thrift, N. (2008b). I just don't know what got into me: Where is the subject?. *Subjectivity, 22*, 82–89.

Thrift, N. (2009). The still point: Resistance, expressive embodiment and dance. In S. Pile & M. Keith (eds.), *Geographies of resistance.* London: Routledge.

Thrift, N., & Dewsbury, J.-D. (2000). Dead geographies–and how to make them live. *Environment and Planning D: Society and Space, 18*, 411–432.

Tomkins, S. (1962). *Affect, imagery and consciousness: The positive affects.* New York: Springer.

Turner, B.S. (1996). *The body and society: Explorations in social theory.* London: Sage.

Uhlmann, A. (1996). To have done with judgement: Beckett and Deleuze. *Substance, 8*, 110–113.

Vahanian, N. (2008). A conversation with Catherine Malabou. *Journal for Cultural and Religious Theory, 9*, 1–13.

REFERENCES 113

Van Huyssteen, J.W. (1999). *The shaping of rationality: Toward interdisciplinarity in theology and science.* Cambridge: Wm. B. Eerdmans.

Vannini, P. (2015). *Non-representational methodologies: Re-envisioning research.* New York: Routledge.

Viveiros De Castro, E. (2012). Intensive filiation and demonic alliance. In Casper B. Jensen & Kjetil Rödje (eds.), *Deleuzian intersections: Science, technology, anthropology.* New York: Berghahn Books.

Voegelin, S. (2014). *Sonic possible worlds: Hearing the continuum of sound.* New York: Bloomsbury.

Waitt, G., Harada, T., & Duffy, M. (2015). 'Let's have some music': Sound, gender and car mobility. *Mobilities.* doi:10.1080/17450101.2015.1076628.

Watson, J. (2009). *Guattari's diagrammatic thought: Writing between Lacan and Deleuze.* London: Continuum.

Whatmore, S. (2002). *Hybrid geographies: Nature, cultures, spaces.* London: Sage.

Whitehead, A.N. (1933). *Adventure of ideas.* New York: The Free Press.

Whitehead, A.N. (1978). *Process and reality (corrected edition).* New York: The Free Press.

Williams, S.J., & Bendelow, G. (1998). *The lived body: Sociological themes, embodied issues.* London: Routledge.

Wittgenstein, L. (1969). *On certainty.* Oxford: Blackwell.

Wylie, J. (2005). A single day's walking: Narrating self and landscape on the South West Coast Path. *Transactions of the Institute of British Geographers, 30,* 234–247.

Young, A. (2014). *Street art, public city: Law, crime and the urban imagination.* London: Routledge.

Yusoff, E. (2014). An interview with Elizabeth Grosz "Ontogenesis and the Ethics of Becoming" by Kathryn Yusoff. *Society and Space Open Journal* (posted 22 May).

Zepke, S. (2005). *Art as abstract machine: Ontology and aesthetics in Deleuze and Guattari.* New York: Routledge.

Zepke, S. (2011). The readymade: Art as the refrain of life. In S. O'Sullivan & S. Zepke (eds.), *Deleuze, Guattari, and the production of the new.* London: Bloomsbury.

INDEX

A

Abstraction, 6, 79, 95

Action, 2, 30–32, 34, 37, 40, 45, 54, 58, 78, 89, 93–95

The actual, 11, 35, 93

Actual occasions, 6

Affect, 2, 5, 14, 19, 22, 34–38, 51, 53, 62, 65, 69, 79, 85, 89

Affective, 2, 21–22, 25, 37, 39, 53, 56, 57, 69, 71, 77, 79, 84, 87–90, 95–96

Affirmation, 5–25, 58

Affirmative, 3, 10, 23, 66

Agency, 2, 8, 20, 30, 31, 34, 54, 93, 94

Assemblages, 17, 20, 22, 23, 30, 31, 34, 35, 69

Atmospheres, 37–38, 62

Attunement, 2, 20, 37, 62, 65, 77–78, 94–95

Audience, 81, 78, 94, 96

Audiencing, 65, 83

Autopoēsis, 23

Avant-garde, 89, 90

B

Becoming, 1, 5, 8, 11–13, 16, 18, 19, 21, 24, 25, 29, 31, 34, 39, 44, 54, 64, 65, 68–71, 89, 91–97

Being, 1, 4, 6, 7, 9, 10–12, 14–17, 19, 21, 24, 25, 30–32, 34, 35, 39, 40, 43, 47, 52, 53, 57, 63, 64, 68, 79, 80, 81–83, 85–87, 94

Bodily, 2, 7, 25, 33, 36, 53, 88, 95

Body, 2, 8–10, 19, 24, 25, 29, 30, 32–37, 44, 46, 51, 56, 57, 62, 64, 66, 68, 69, 79, 81, 82, 85, 92, 94, 95

C

Capacities, 5, 9, 21, 24, 32, 33, 36, 52, 57, 62, 79, 82, 83, 94, 96

Change and transformation, 1, 17, 96

Context, 2, 20, 22, 31, 36, 48–51, 62, 92–93, 95, 96

Creativity, 7, 10, 21, 22, 44, 79, 82

© The Author(s) 2017

C.P. Boyd, *Non-Representational Geographies of Therapeutic Art Making*, DOI 10.1007/978-3-319-46286-8

116 INDEX

D
Dancing, 49, 54, 63, 67–70, 80
Desiring-production, 11, 35, 80
De-territorialisaiton, 21, 23, 25, 66, 79, 81
Difference, 11, 12, 17, 20, 21, 33, 47, 51, 81, 92
Drawing, 29, 30, 37, 62, 63, 67–70, 84
Duration, 12, 57, 83, 68, 87–89

E
Ekphrasis, 62, 63, 66, 67, 76–78, 89
Ekphrastic, 61–90
Ethical, 20, 24, 25, 48, 56, 58, 67, 92, 93, 97
Ethico-aesthetic, 1, 20–22, 68, 79, 96
Ethics, 3, 5–25
Ethnographic, 44, 58
Ethnography, 44
Event, 6, 7, 11–14, 18, 19, 22, 24, 27–29, 31, 33, 48, 54, 84, 63–69, 79, 80, 88, 91, 93, 96
Experience, 1, 3, 4, 7–10, 14–16, 18, 24–25, 29, 33–35, 37–39, 48–50, 52–54, 62–66, 80, 84, 78, 92–96
Experiment, 3, 22, 23, 35, 48, 51, 54, 56, 62, 64–66, 68, 80, 83, 84, 87, 94
Extension, 3, 6, 9, 12, 13, 20, 62, 70, 92
Extensive, 37, 39

F
Feeling, 6, 25, 32, 36, 37, 40, 54–57, 64, 70, 78, 95, 96
Fibre art, 44, 50
Fielding, 94–95

Fieldwork, 3, 44, 50, 52, 54–57, 62, 67, 68, 83, 88, 94
Film, 45, 48, 49, 50, 55, 57, 85, 87–90

G
General Assembly, 50, 51
Graffiti, 49–50, 81, 91
Grounding, 69, 70

H
Habit, 9, 30, 37, 57, 85

I
Intensity, 11, 12, 14, 20, 36, 37, 63, 96
Intensive, 5, 39, 54, 87, 93
Intersubjectivity, 9, 58

J
Joint Action, 30–32, 94

K
Knowledge, 3, 8, 28, 33, 37, 45–47, 50–52, 56, 57, 61, 67, 69, 70, 78, 90, 94, 95–96

L
Lines of flight, 21, 79, 96

M
Mapping, 63, 70–80
Materiality, 17, 19–20, 31, 32, 34–35, 38–40, 50, 64, 65, 89, 93–94

INDEX 117

Matter, 13, 18, 20, 23, 29, 30, 32, 33, 62, 65, 93
Memory, 41, 44, 48, 50, 54, 55, 57–59, 64, 65, 85
Methodology, 3, 29, 38, 43, 44, 57, 59, 67
Montage, 63, 78–90
Movement, 2, 29, 30, 32, 34, 35, 38, 44, 49, 51, 55, 58, 63, 67, 62, 63, 65, 68–72, 83, 78–89, 92
Multiplicity, 11–12, 89
Music, 46, 51, 62, 63, 67–69, 83, 85, 78

N
Neo-avant-garde, 89
New materialism, 17
Nomadic, 24
Non-human, 1, 2, 19, 20, 30, 38, 45, 54, 55, 62, 82, 83, 88, 92–94
Non-representational theory, 2, 3, 5, 23, 27–41, 43, 49, 56, 95

O
Object-oriented ontology, 17, 56
Ontic, 19, 93–94
Ontological, 10, 12, 13, 17, 18, 20, 78, 94
Openness, 8, 15, 20, 36, 61, 79, 85

P
Painting, 14, 48, 49, 50, 54, 62, 63–67, 70–80, 84, 88, 90, 93
Perception, 7–10, 22, 24, 32, 34, 36, 52, 57, 62, 88, 92, 95
Performative research paradigm, 44–47
Phenomenology, 13, 18

Photography, 49, 54–55, 82, 83, 78–90
Poetic permaculture, 44, 49, 81
Poetry, 62, 63–67, 84
Post-human, 33, 62
Post-phenomenology, 13
Post-structural, 8, 34, 91
Potential, 1, 2, 5, 6, 11, 13, 18, 20, 22, 24, 33, 39, 45, 53, 56, 57, 59, 66, 69, 79, 96
Practice-led, 3, 44–48
Practice-based, 3, 44, 46, 49, 50
Pre-cognitive, 32–33, 64, 93
Prehension, 6
Proprioception, 53

R
Refrain, 23, 50, 65, 92
Representational, 2, 16
Research-creation, 44, 53, 54, 56, 59
Re-territorialisation, 21, 81

S
Saturated phenomena, 14, 64
Schizoanalysis, 63, 80
Schizoanalytic, 23, 48, 63, 70–80
Self, 2, 3, 11, 12, 14–16, 23–25, 31, 32, 44, 50, 52, 57–59, 66, 79, 78, 93, 96
Senses, 6, 25, 52, 53, 62, 82, 91–92
Sensing, 1, 3, 8, 25, 33, 34, 39, 51, 53, 54, 56, 68, 92, 93
Sensory, 8, 14, 25, 92, 94
Social, 2, 4, 9, 21, 22, 27, 28, 31, 33–40, 48, 53, 62, 79, 80, 94, 95
Soundscape, 49, 50, 80–84, 89
Space, 1, 2, 4, 8, 23, 27, 31, 34, 35, 38–41, 51–53, 55, 63, 64, 74–78, 88, 91–93, 95, 96

118 INDEX

Spacings, 39, 54–57
Speculative realism, 5, 18, 19
Stop-frame animation, 84, 63, 87–89
Subjectivation, 16, 21–23, 30,
    79, 80, 88
Subjectivity, 2, 8–10, 12, 13, 20–23,
    30, 38, 39, 58, 79
Super, 8, 48, 49, 63, 69, 89, 90
Synaesthetic, 38, 92

T
Techniques, 4, 29, 54, 62–63, 83, 84,
    85, 90, 94, 95
Testimony, 52, 53, 57

Therapeutic space, 1, 2, 13, 84, 93
Translation, 56, 90, 95–96
Transversal, 3, 4, 21,
    22, 64, 79, 93

V
The virtual, 11, 12, 22, 35, 36, 66, 70,
    79, 87, 93, 97
Vital materialism, 17–18, 20

W
Witnessing, 52, 68, 95
Wonder, 25, 55, 69, 84, 97

Printed in the United States
By Bookmasters